thefacts

Cystic
fibrosis

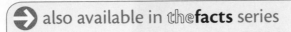

also available in the**facts** series

the**facts**

Cystic fibrosis

FULLY UPDATED AND REVISED
FOURTH EDITION

ANNE H THOMSON
Director, Oxford Paediatric Cystic Fibrosis Centre, Oxford
Children's Hospital

ANN HARRIS
Director, Human Molecular Genetics Program, Children's
Memorial Research Center, Northwestern University Feinberg
School of Medicine

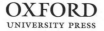

OXFORD
UNIVERSITY PRESS

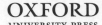
OXFORD
UNIVERSITY PRESS

Great Clarendon Street, Oxford OX2 6DP

Oxford University Press is a department of the University of Oxford.
It furthers the University's objective of excellence in research, scholarship,
and education by publishing worldwide in

Oxford New York

Auckland Cape Town Dar es Salaam Hong Kong Karachi
Kuala Lumpur Madrid Melbourne Mexico City Nairobi
New Delhi Shanghai Taipei Toronto

With offices in

Argentina Austria Brazil Chile Czech Republic France Greece
Guatemala Hungary Italy Japan Poland Portugal Singapore
South Korea Switzerland Thailand Turkey Ukraine Vietnam

Oxford is a registered trade mark of Oxford University Press
in the UK and in certain other countries

Published in the United States
by Oxford University Press Inc., New York

British Library Cataloguing in Publication Data

Data available

Library of Congress Cataloging-in-Publication Data

Thomson, Anne H.
  Cystic fibrosis: the facts / Anne H. Thomson, Ann Harris. — 4th ed.
  p. cm. — (the facts)
  ISBN 978–0–19–929580–7
1. Cystic fibrosis—Popular works. I. Harris, Ann. II. Title.
  RC858.C95T56 2008
  616.3′72—dc22

                                                                    2008017227

ISBN 978–0–19–929580–7

1 3 5 7 9 10 8 6 4 2

Typeset in Plantin
by Cepha Imaging Pvt. Ltd., Bangalore, India
Printed in China
by Asia Pacific Offset

Preface

It is now more than 20 years since the first edition of *Cystic Fibrosis: The Facts* was published, two years before the gene that causes CF was identified. Two subsequent editions, both co-authored by Maurice Super, were published in 1990 and 1995. During the past 20 years there have been many advances in the treatment of CF and the median survival rate has increased by about 10 years. With increased survival, new aspects of the disease need to be dealt with and the growth of adult CF clinics has changed the emphasis of CF care from a mainly paediatric specialty to both childhood and adult medicine.

Cystic Fibrosis: The Facts 2008 edition is completely rewritten and takes a new approach to the disease and its treatment, with up-to-date information on all aspects of life with CF. One chapter that cannot yet be written describes an effective cure for the disease. Many research scientists and physicians are working hard to achieve this, but we cannot predict when it will become a reality. In the meantime we hope that this book is helpful to all those who encounter CF in their lives.

Oxford	A.H.T
Chicago	A.H.
May 2008	

Acknowledgements

The authors would like to thank many people for their contributions to this book:

First, and most importantly, the young people and their parents who have shared their experiences with us. Also Dr Bee Brockman for illustrations and Dr Konrad Jacobs, Dr Louisa Demetriades, and Dr Julian Forton for contributing chapters. Finally our colleagues whose discussions and comments over many years have helped our understanding of this complex disease.

The authors thank Dr Susanna McColley, Director of the Cystic Fibrosis Center at Children's Memorial Hospital, Chicago for her valuable input on differences in cystic fibrosis care in the UK and the USA.

Contents

1

Introduction and making the diagnosis

→ Key points

- Cystic fibrosis (CF) occurs when a person has inherited two copies of a faulty gene (one from each parent)
- CF is suspected in children who:

    (a) have a bowel blockage at birth

    (b) fail to gain weight even when eating well

    (c) have frequent smelly stools

    (d) have a persistent or recurrent wet cough or chest infection

- Newborn infants can now be screened for CF by a heel-prick blood test

- The diagnosis of CF is confirmed by a sweat test which measures the concentration of chloride (as salt) in the sweat

What is cystic fibrosis?

Cystic fibrosis is a disease caused when a person has inherited two copies of a faulty gene (one from each parent). The disease can affect many parts of the body but most importantly involves the lungs and the gut. The problem in the lungs causes difficulty in clearing secretions (mucus), and in the gut causes difficulty in absorbing food properly. This book is written for families, friends, teachers and all those who encounter CF in their lives. It tries to explain the disease, its management and how it affects individuals.

Why is it called cystic fibrosis?

The name comes from changes in a gland called the pancreas. The pancreas makes enzymes that help digest food and some other compounds. It is damaged from early life in most people with cystic fibrosis and is gradually replaced with scar tissue (fibrosis) and fluid-filled spaces (cysts). Cystic fibrosis was only recognized as a distinct disorder in 1938.

When is cystic fibrosis suspected?

Cystic fibrosis has traditionally been suspected in young children who were either failing to gain weight (failing to thrive) even when eating well or had persistent or recurrent chest infections. Some infants have problems at birth with blockage (obstruction) of the bowel (meconium ileus). Less commonly children come to medical attention with other bowel symptoms or symptoms of nasal obstruction (nasal polyps). Occasionally cystic fibrosis is diagnosed in adult men presenting with infertility. However, increasingly in many countries children are being diagnosed with cystic fibrosis as a result of being screened for the disease at birth. Neonatal screening for cystic fibrosis became universal in England in 2007, and is available in some US states.

Newborn screening

There are minor variations in national screening programmes. In England the screening is done on blood spots taken from the infant (on day five or six) on the Guthrie card. The blood is first checked for the level of an enzyme called immunoreactive trypsin (IRT). If the level is much higher than normal the blood is then checked for the common cystic fibrosis mutations. If two mutations are found then the child is presumed to have cystic fibrosis and is referred to a cystic fibrosis centre to confirm the diagnosis. If only one cystic fibrosis mutation is found then a second blood sample is taken between days 21 and 28 for a further measurement of immunoreactive trypsin. If this level is also high then the child is likely to have cystic fibrosis and is referred to the cystic fibrosis centre for confirmation of the diagnosis. If the level is low the child is likely not to have cystic fibrosis but carries one cystic fibrosis mutation, that is, they are a carrier for cystic fibrosis.

In the United States, newborn screening programmes are run at the state rather than national level. All programmes use similar techniques. The initial blood spot is taken at one to two days of age and tested for IRT. Some states perform tests for cystic fibrosis gene mutations on all samples with an elevated IRT, while others measure a second IRT instead. Another variation is to perform

Table 1.1 Frequency of symptoms in cystic fibrosis

Failure to gain weight	43%
Persistent wet cough/Recurrent chest infections	51%
Smelly fatty stools	35%
Meconium ileus	18%
Family history (no symptoms)	16%

genetic testing after a second IRT is found to be elevated. Because genetic testing is usually limited to the most common gene mutations causing CF, and because of the genetic diversity of the population in the US, tests are considered positive even if only one CF mutation is found. This means that all infants with elevated IRT and one or two CF gene mutations are referred for sweat testing. In some states, a very high (sometimes called 'ultra high') IRT is also considered to be a positive newborn screen for CF, prompting sweat testing.

Most children diagnosed by newborn screening will be entirely well at the time that the diagnosis is made. Once newborn screening is universally available it is likely that very few children will present with the other symptoms described above (Table 1.1).

Failure to thrive

The child with cystic fibrosis is usually hungry for food and eats well. However, because the food is not absorbed properly it passes through the bowel, giving frequent smelly loose stools which may look slimy or greasy. This is called steatorrhoea. The stools contain lots of globules of fat.

Chest infection

All young children are exposed to viral infections and coughs with colds are frequent. However, suspicions of cystic fibrosis are raised if the cough does not clear between viral infections and in particular if it sounds as if there is mucus present (a smoker's cough).

Meconium ileus

Approximately 15 per cent of children with cystic fibrosis will present soon after birth with bowel obstruction. The infant may start to vomit, the abdomen becomes distended and no stool is passed. An x-ray of the abdomen confirms bowel obstruction and in most cases an attempt to clear the bowel is made by passing a dye-containing substance (gastrografin) up as an enema into the bowel. If this does not clear the obstruction then surgery may be necessary.

The first stool that a newborn baby passes is a sticky black motion and is called meconium. In cystic fibrosis the meconium is stickier than normal and sometimes does not pass all the way through the bowel but gets stuck, often at the junction between the small and the large bowel, causing the obstruction.

At surgery the bowel is opened at the site of obstruction and the sticky meconium removed. In many cases the surgeon will be able to join the bowel together again, but sometimes this is not possible and a loop of bowel is brought through the skin to form an ileostomy. The ileostomy is temporary and is usually closed after a few weeks.

The finding of meconium ileus is highly suggestive of cystic fibrosis as the underlying diagnosis (greater than 95 per cent). The diagnosis is later confirmed as described below.

Rectal prolapse

This occurs when a small part of the lining of the bowel protrudes through the anus after a child has passed stool. It is most likely to occur in a child who is passing large bulky stools with effort. It is most common therefore in constipation, but can occur in cystic fibrosis.

Nasal polyps

Nasal polyps are not very common in children but sometimes occur in children who are very allergic and have lots of hay fever-type symptoms. They can also occur in cystic fibrosis and very rarely they are what brings the child with cystic fibrosis to medical attention.

Infertility

The man with cystic fibrosis lacks parts of the small tube in which sperm travel down from the testes (the vas deferens). Men who are mildly affected by cystic fibrosis may have no other symptoms and the diagnosis is made when they go to an infertility clinic. (This is explained fully in Chapter 14.)

How is the diagnosis of cystic fibrosis confirmed?

The standard test for the diagnosis of cystic fibrosis is a sweat test. Individuals with cystic fibrosis have much higher concentrations of sodium and chloride (salt) in their sweat than normal.

The sweat test is most commonly done on the forearm. The first step is to stimulate sweating by placing two pads containing a special medicine called pilocarpine on the forearm and by using a small electrical current from a battery to drive the medicine in through the skin. The pads are then removed and the skin cleaned. A special sweat-collecting device is then placed on the forearm (Figure 1.1) and the sweat collected over the next 30 minutes. The sweat is then analysed for chloride content. A sweat chloride greater than 60 mmols/litre is diagnostic of cystic fibrosis in children. Normal sweat chloride levels are lower in newborns and higher in adults, so slightly different sweat chloride levels are used to make a diagnosis of cystic fibrosis in these age groups.

Can there be problems with the sweat test?

The test needs to be done carefully by an experienced operator. The most common problem is that the child does not sweat enough. It is important for

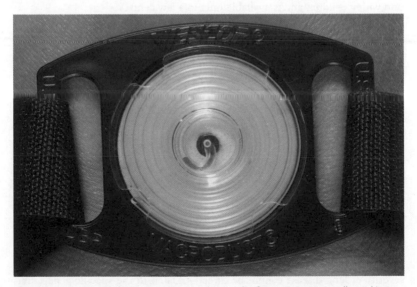

Figure 1.1 A macroduct sweat-collecting disc on the forearm. Sweat is collected in a small capillary tube within the disc.

the accuracy of the test that a certain amount of sweat is collected within the 30-minute period. If there is insufficient sweat then the test will need to be repeated on another day.

Can the diagnosis of cystic fibrosis be made genetically?

Yes. If the child has two cystic fibrosis mutations then the diagnosis is confirmed. However, the usual laboratory tests will only detect about 30 of the most common genetic mutations so will make the diagnosis in only about 75 per cent of cases. As over 1500 mutations causing cystic fibrosis have been identified it is possible for the usual laboratory test to miss a rare mutation. For this reason the sweat test is still used as 'the gold standard'. It is now possible to look for all the known mutations in the cystic fibrosis gene, but this is both very costly and takes some months for results to be available.

Are there any other tests used in diagnosis?

Very rarely it is impossible to confirm the diagnosis by either genetics or sweat test. A sophisticated test on cells lining the nose, called nasal potential difference, can be used to give additional information. This test can be difficult in infants and young children and is available only in a few centres.

There can also be other helpful information. For example the stool can be examined for fat and for a pancreatic enzyme called elastase. A low stool elastase level confirms that the pancreas is not working properly (pancreatic insufficiency). There are rare occasions when all the tests are inconclusive and the cystic fibrosis specialist has to put all the information together and decide whether the individual has cystic fibrosis on the balance of probabilities. The diagnosis is usually confirmed with time.

Will my child have mild or severe cystic fibrosis symptoms?

It is impossible to say how severe CF disease will be in any individual but some general statements can be made. Some gene mutations such as the commonest, *delta F508* (ΔF508), (See Chapter 13) are almost always associated with the need for pancreatic supplements. Individuals with combinations of some other genes such as *R117H* and *S1251N* will rarely need pancreatic supplements. The severity of lung disease cannot be directly related to the specific gene mutation and it is clear that many other things including nutrition, environmental exposure to pollutants including cigarette smoke, viral infections and the rest of a person's genetic make-up determines how severe their lung disease is. It is also probable that other genetic variations between individuals can affect disease severity (see Chapter 13).

 ## Patient's perspective

Katherine had been worried about her baby Robert since he was a few weeks old. Although he initially breastfed well and put on weight, after a few weeks the breast no longer seemed to satisfy him and he had both breast and bottle feeds. He passed soft, rather slimy stools four or five times a day and they smelt. Family members joked that you could tell he needed a nappy change from the room next door. However, he was 3 months old when he had his first bad cold and developed a cough that would not clear. After three visits to the family doctor Robert was referred to a paediatrician.

At the clinic visit, the doctor noted that despite having a good intake of bottle milk plus additional breastfeeds Roberts weight had fallen from the middle line on the growth chart (50th centile) at birth to just above the bottom line (3rd centile). He was bright and alert but looked a little scrawny and had a productive-sounding cough. The paediatrician arranged for a sample of his stool to be examined for fat and for elastase measurement and for a sweat test to be done.

The sweat test showed a high sweat-chloride level, confirming the diagnosis of cystic fibrosis. The stool sample showed a large excess of fat globules and the elastase level was low, confirming pancreatic insufficiency.

Robert was started on one half capsule of Creon per feed and Katherine was delighted to find that within 3 days his stools were completely different and he did not seem so hungry. On treatment with antibiotics and physiotherapy his cough cleared in 10 days.

2

How cystic fibrosis affects the lungs

> **→ Key points**
>
> ◆ Mucus in the lungs is cleared less efficiently in CF
>
> ◆ Bacteria can settle on the surface of the airways (infection) and cause inflammation and increased mucus production
>
> ◆ Regular monitoring with cough swabs or sputum samples will pick up bacterial infection early
>
> ◆ Simple blowing tests (lung function tests) are used to monitor lung health

The lung consists of airways and air spaces. The major airway is called the trachea and this then divides into airways (the bronchi) to the right and to the left lung. The airways then continue to divide, getting smaller and smaller as they get towards the periphery of the lung. Each tiny airway, now called a bronchiole, leads into a collection of air sacs called alveoli (Figure 2.1). The air sacs are surrounded by blood vessels and, as we breathe, oxygen passes from the air sacs into the bloodstream and hence is delivered to the body tissues. The waste product carbon dioxide (CO_2) passes back from the bloodstream into the air sacs and is breathed out.

Each airway in the lung is lined with cells which have on their surface small hairs called cilia. These cilia move within a liquid lining the airway surface (airway surface liquid) and the cilia tips project into the mucus produced by the airways (Figure 2.2). The cilia beat in a rhythmical fashion to move mucus up the airways to the back of the throat where it is swallowed.

The air that we breathe contains tiny particles of debris and bacteria. This generally lands on the mucus of the airways, and as the mucus is continuously

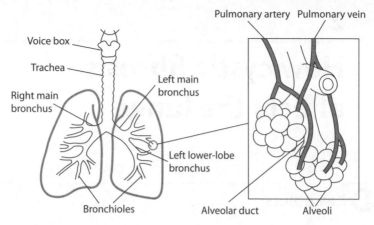

Figure 2.1 A diagram of the lungs.

moved up the airways by the cilia so the debris and bacteria are cleared from the lung.

The abnormality in cystic fibrosis results in the liquid layer, in which the cilia beat, being smaller (less deep) (Figure 2.3). This means that the cilia are not able to work as efficiently, so mucus is not cleared from the lungs as effectively and bacteria are not cleared from the lungs as efficiently. In addition, when bacteria are present, there seems to be an increased amount of inflammation produced in the lung in cystic fibrosis. It is not yet understood why this is so.

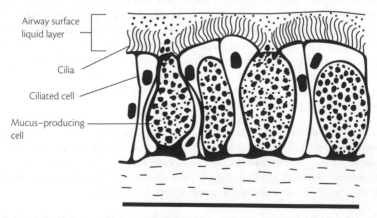

Figure 2.2 A diagram of the airway surface.

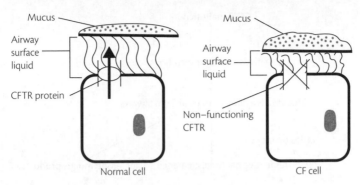

Figure 2.3 A normal airway cell and an airway cell in cystic fibrosis showing the decreased depth of the liquid layer surrounding the cilia. The arrow shows normal salt and water movement through the CFTR.

All children will get coughs and colds with viral infections – on average a pre-school child will get between 6 and 12 viral infections per year. A child with cystic fibrosis is no more likely than others to get a viral infection. However, viral respiratory infections result in increased mucus production and, as described above, children with cystic fibrosis are less efficient at clearing mucus from the chest. Children with cystic fibrosis therefore tend to have chest problems for longer with viral infections and, at a time when there is increased mucus around and decreased clearance of any bacteria that are present, they are more likely to get a secondary infection with a bacterium. This is why children and adults with cystic fibrosis are advised to start antibiotic treatment when they have increased respiratory symptoms with colds even though we know the cold is caused by a virus.

What happens when there is a bacterial growth in the airways?

If the bacteria settle on the surface of the airways and are not cleared effectively they multiply and cause inflammation and increased mucus production (see Chapter 8). The normal cells lining the airways are damaged. If there is prompt treatment with antibiotics and the bacteria are killed then the normal cells lining the airways will repair themselves. However, over time and with repeated infection there may be permanent inflammation and thickening of the airway walls. Eventually this can lead to blockage of some of the very smallest airways and dilatation of others, with permanent mucus over-production and an inability to completely clear bacterial infection (Figure 2.4).

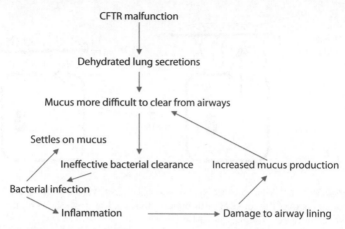

Figure 2.4 The cycle of infection, airway damage, increased mucous production and ineffective clearance of bacteria.

How does lung disease in cystic fibrosis progress?

As the small airways become partially blocked air can reach the air sacs (alveoli) during inspiration – breathing in, which is when the small airways expand – but the air may not be able to leave during expiration – breathing out – thus leading to air trapping and over-inflation of that area of the lung. This over-inflation increases with time, and if it is happening in many areas of the lung it may result in the chest looking over-expanded, with an increase in the depth of the chest from breastbone to back. In addition chronic infection in the smallest airways leads to dilatation of the airway such that it becomes a rounded structure in cross-section (cyst-like) with collection of infected mucus inside. This is known as bronchiectasis. As over-inflation and bronchiectasis increase, the ability of the lung to exchange gases decreases. This means that the lungs cannot transfer oxygen to, and have difficulty clearing carbon dioxide from, the bloodstream.

How is lung disease monitored?

The doctor will examine the child's chest regularly and may be able to pick up signs of infection or over inflation. The child is likely to have a chest radiograph (chest x-ray) at least once a year and more often if they are having infections. However, the chest x-ray is only a crude guide to what is happening in the lung (Figure 2.5) The most important tests are lung function or breathing tests. Once a child reaches the age of 5 or 6 years they will be taught how to do lung function tests. This generally involves the child taking a deep

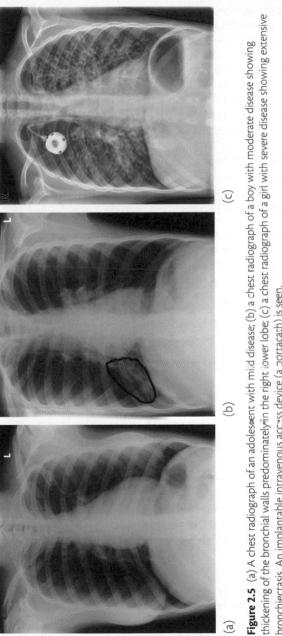

(a)

(b)

(c)

Figure 2.5 (a) A chest radiograph of an adolescent with mild disease; (b) a chest radiograph of a boy with moderate disease showing thickening of the bronchial walls predominately in the right lower lobe; (c) a chest radiograph of a girl with severe disease showing extensive bronchiectasis. An implantable intravenous access device (a portacath) is seen.

breath and then blowing out into a machine as fast and as hard as they can. To get good results needs maximum effort and it may take some time before the young child is able to do the tests satisfactorily. These tests are called spirometry (Figure 2.6). A number of measurements can be made from these tests but the most widely used are the Forced Vital Capacity (FVC) – the total volume of air blown out; the Forced Expiratory Volume (FEV_1) – the volume of air blown out in the first second; and an assessment of the shape of the loop that is produced when the volume of air that is blown out is plotted on a graph against the rate at which the air flows out from the lungs (the flow–volume loop) (Figure 2.7). The FVC and the FEV_1 can be compared with standard values for children of the same age, sex and height. These measurements can be done at each clinic visit and changes noted over time.

Other less frequent tests

More sophisticated lung function tests which can measure the amount of over-inflation usually involve a visit to a lung function laboratory and are done less often, perhaps once a year. Sometimes a test called a ventilation scan can be useful. This is when a special gas which has a small amount of radioactivity is breathed in, and a special camera can show where the gas goes to in the lungs. If there is a part of the lung where the airways are blocked then the gas can't get in and this shows on the scan. Unfortunately these scans can sometimes be

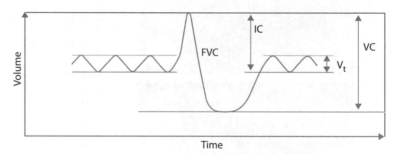

Figure 2.6 Lung function assessment. Technique: the child is asked to breath normally then to take as big a breath as they can and then to blow out as fast and hard as they can and to keep going until their lungs are completely empty of air. The plot is of volume of air against time, showing three normal breaths in and out followed by a large breath in, a large breath out and then two more normal breaths.

FVC = forced vital capacity (the volume of air that can be forcibly blown out); IC = inspiratory capacity (the maximum volume of air that can be breathed in); V_t = tidal volume (the volume of air breathed in with each normal breath); VC = vital capacity (the maximum volume of air that can be held in the lungs).

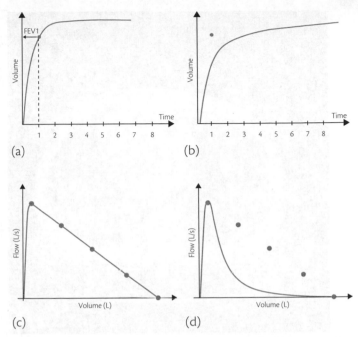

Figure 2.7 Lung function tests. (a) Shows a plot of the volume of air blown out against the time taken to blow out. With normal lungs nearly all the air is blown out in the first second. The FEV_1 is the volume of air blown out in the first second. The FVC is the total volume of air blown out. (b) Shows what happens with severe lung disease in cystic fibrosis. It takes much longer to blow the air out and the total volume of air is also reduced. (c) Shows the rate of air flow plotted against the volume blown out. This is called the expiratory flow–volume loop. With normal lungs the shape is near to a triangle. (d) Shows a flow–volume loop taken during an exacerbation of lung disease in cystic fibrosis. The flow rates are much lower throughout the blow and the shape becomes scooped out.

too sensitive so that there can be big changes, for example after physiotherapy. Another type of scan called a computerized tomography (CT) scan is used if there is concern about a person's lungs or a particular part of the lung (Figure 2.8). A CT scan can show in detail the structure of the airways and air spaces, including early bronchiectasis, by recording x-ray images that slice through the lungs. A standard child CT scan involves a much higher radiation dose than a chest x-ray (approximately 100 times) and so the dose is reduced by using only selected slices through the lung. CT scans are often used for monitoring in research studies and increasingly in selected cases where there is a problem. It is likely that in the future the techniques will improve to decrease the amount of radiation used and CT scanning will be more frequent.

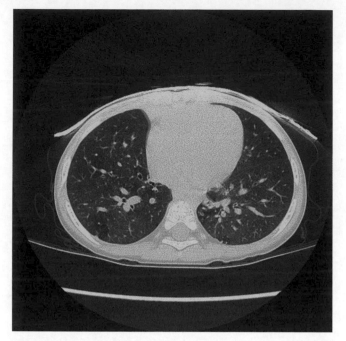

Figure 2.8 A CT scan image showing early bronchiectasis.

Chest infection in cystic fibrosis

Health and survival in cystic fibrosis are clearly related to the presence, the severity and the progress of chest infection. The main objective in treatment is to prevent, clear or control all types of respiratory infection.

 FAQ

How can I tell if my child is developing a chest infection?

All children will get colds and coughs but these are taken more seriously in cystic fibrosis. If your child has a cold and starts coughing then take action. Increase the frequency of physiotherapy and if your child is on preventive antibiotics then increase them, for example from twice daily to four times a day. If there is no improvement in 2 days or if they are becoming more unwell then contact your doctor or CF nurse for advice and to arrange a cough swab/sputum sample. An alternative antibiotic may be started. Early warning signs of an infection are given in Table 2.1.

Table 2.1 Early warning signs of an infection/exacerbation

Increased cough
Increased sputum
Change in sputum appearance
Fever
Decreased appetite
Difficulty breathing
Decreased exercise ability

Is it viruses or bacteria that are important in cystic fibrosis?

It is important to remember that we all carry many bacteria in our bodies, on our skin, in our throat and in our gut. For the most part we live happily with them. People with cystic fibrosis are no different. However, bacteria which we carry in our throat can freely move into the lung with breathing, especially if our natural defences are disrupted. Viral infections such as the common cold disrupt natural defences by damaging the surfaces of cells lining the airways and therefore bacteria carried in the throat are more likely to enter the lower airways at this time. Bacteria are more difficult to clear in cystic fibrosis. It is for this reason that doctors advise early treatment with antibiotics in people with cystic fibrosis, even if the symptoms start with a cold. This can cause confusion as antibiotics do not work for virus infections but do act against the secondary bacterial invader. Some viruses themselves cause lower airway symptoms, for example influenza, and can cause more severe infections in the cystic fibrosis lung. For details of specific bacteria see Chapter 8.

Can infection be prevented?

All children and adults with cystic fibrosis will get infections. It is possible however to take some precautions to avoid unnecessary infection. First, infants

Table 2.2 Avoiding infection

Cover the mouth and nose when you cough or sneeze
Wash your hands a lot
Do not share cups, cans or bottles
Do not share physio equipment or nebulizing equipment
Know which bacteria you most often carry

and children with cystic fibrosis should have all the normal immunizations. In addition they should have flu vaccination each year. It is clear that bacterial infection often follows a viral infection and so where possible infants and young children should avoid close contact with individuals who have colds.

There are some infections which can be transmitted between cystic fibrosis patients. Individuals with cystic fibrosis should therefore avoid close personal contact such as kissing or sharing eating utensils with other non-family members who have cystic fibrosis (Table 2.2). Hospital services are very aware of the possibility of cross-infection between patients. Patients with resistant organisms are kept separate from other patients. It is important to remember that many organisms which cause problems in CF are environmental organisms and most infections are required incidentally in the community. Normal public swimming pools have high standards of infection control and are safe for people with cystic fibrosis, but many bugs thrive in warm wet conditions so jacuzzis should be avoided.

How can the lungs be kept clear?

Clearing mucus from the airways is a very important part of cystic fibrosis preventative management. Exercise and physiotherapy are the main strategies and the techniques are expanded on in Chapter 5.

Other lung complications

Wheezing and asthma

A large number of children and adults with cystic fibrosis wheeze at times, particularly with viral infections. In some this may be because they, by chance, also have asthma but in others it may simply be as a result of airway inflammation related to their cystic fibrosis. It is usually worthwhile trying inhaled bronchodilators (as used in asthma) and many patients do respond. It is less clear how often inhaled steroid therapy is useful in cystic fibrosis.

Allergic bronchopulmonary aspergillosis (ABPA)

This is where the body develops an allergic response to an inhaled fungal organism – *Aspergillus*. It occurs in about one in 20 patients with cystic fibrosis. *Aspergillus* is a common organism found particularly in hay, rotting compost or other vegetable matter, and in old buildings. It can be released into the air during building work. Sometimes it will settle on the airways and provoke an allergic response causing wheezing and a fall in lung function. The allergic response can be picked up on blood tests and one of these tests – the total IgE level – is used to monitor the effects of treatment. There can be characteristic fluffy shadows seen on the chest radiograph (x-ray) in some (but not all) people who have ABPA. Treatment is with steroids to control the allergic response and antifungal drugs such as itraconazole.

Haemoptysis (coughing up blood)

Blood streaking of the sputum is common particularly in older patients and is often associated with an infection. Coughing up larger amounts of blood can occur as the disease progresses when a small blood vessel ruptures into an airspace. Most often this settles but occasionally surgery is needed.

Pneumothorax

This is when a small bleb on the surface of the lung bursts, releasing air into a space between the lung and the chest wall hence causing partial collapse of the lung. In cystic fibrosis this is most likely to occur in older patients with severe lung disease and one in five individuals will experience this in their life. A drain placed through the chest wall into the space between the chest wall and the lung is usually required to suck out the air and allow the lung to re-expand.

Nasal polyps

Children and adults with cystic fibrosis are more likely to develop nasal polyps. These are outgrowths of the mucous membranes and seem to be a response of the nasal mucosa to irritation or infection. Nasal polyps are also common in people with allergies. Nasal steroid sprays will shrink polyps and are often sufficient treatment. Some individuals need surgery to remove the polyps and then use steroids to prevent recurrence.

Patient's perspective

Christine was 10 years old and had been diagnosed with cystic fibrosis at 3 months of age as a result of poor weight gain and smelly stools. She had been well and had little trouble with her chest until April when she had started with a dry-sounding cough. As this was unusual her mother arranged for a cough swab to be done and while waiting the results she was started on the antibiotic flucloxacillin.

The cough swab did not grow any organisms but the cough persisted and Christine started to produce a little white phlegm. A sample of the phlegm was obtained for culture and in the meantime the antibiotic was changed to one which covered a broad spectrum of organisms. Once again there was no growth from the culture. Christine felt her cough was a bit better but noticed she was getting a little breathless on exercise, which had never happened before.

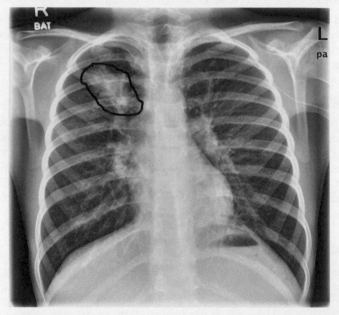

Figure 2.9 A chest x-ray showing the fluffy shadow of allergic bronchopulmonary aspergillosis.

When Christine saw the CF specialist he arranged for a chest radiograph (chest x-ray) to be done and noted that at Christine's annual review 10 months before she had shown some evidence of sensitivity to *Aspergillus*, with a raised specific *Aspergillus* IgE titre. He arranged for this blood test to be repeated along with a total IgE level.

The chest x-ray showed a fluffy shadow in keeping with an allergic response to *Aspergillus* (allergic bronchopulmonary aspergillosis or ABPA) (Figure 2.9) and Christine was started on some treatment with daily steroid tablets (prednisolone). When seen for review 2 weeks later she was much better and her blood test results confirmed a very high total IgE level in keeping with the diagnosis of ABPA.

3

How cystic fibrosis affects the digestive system

➔ Key points

♦ The pancreas is the gland which produces enzymes to digest foodstuffs

♦ All individuals with CF produce decreased amounts of enzymes

♦ Around 85 per cent of people with CF cannot produce enough enzymes for efficient digestion and absorption of food and need to take additional enzymes by mouth with each meal

♦ Around 15 per cent of babies with CF have blockage of the bowel from birth; this is called meconium ileus

Normal digestion

Food is broken down from complex proteins, fats and carbohydrates to simple molecules of amino acids, fatty acids and sugars which can be absorbed through the walls of the small intestine into the bloodstream. These are then transported by the bloodstream to the liver where further metabolism takes place.

Proteins

Proteins are made of long chains of amino acids and are first broken down into short chains (peptides) and then to individual amino acids. Amino acids are essential for tissue growth and repair and to replace cells as they die.

Fats

Fats are broken down into glycerol and fatty acids. Fatty acids are essential in the formation of cell membranes. Fats are important for energy storage.

Carbohydrates

Carbohydrates are starches and consist of long chains of complex sugars (polysaccharides). These are broken down to shorter and shorter chains and eventually to simple sugars (glucose, fructose and galactose). Glucose is the main body fuel and ready glucose energy is stored in the liver and in the muscles as glycogen.

The digestive tract

In the mouth food is broken down and mixed with saliva which contains an enzyme (amylase) that starts the digestion of carbohydrates. After being swallowed food travels down the gullet (oesophagus) to the stomach (Figure 3.1). The stomach produces hydrochloric acid and the enzyme pepsin which breaks down proteins to peptides. The presence of food in the stomach stimulates the production of a hormone which in turn stimulates the production of digestive juices by the pancreas. A bolus of food passes from the stomach into the duodenum (the first part of the small intestine). Pancreatic secretions containing bicarbonate and the digestive enzymes lipase, amylase and trypsin are released into the duodenum through the pancreatic duct, and bile salts from the liver also mix here. Trypsin completes the breakdown of peptides to amino acids; amylase continues the breakdown of carbohydrates; and fats are emulsified by the bile salts and then broken down by lipase to glycerol and fatty acids.

The food bolus continues to move slowly through the small intestine (the jejunum and then the ileum). The surface of the small intestine consists of small finger-like protrusions (villi) which increase the surface area available for food absorption. The amino acids, sugars and fatty acids are absorbed into the bloodstream and transported to the liver. Substances which cannot be digested, such as fibre and other waste products, stay in the small intestine and pass in to the caecum which is a mixing chamber at the start of the large intestine. Bacteria are normally present in the caecum and act on the waste products to break them down by a process of fermentation. This fermentation also results in the formation of gas (flatus or wind). If there is poor absorption of food, especially fat, this process of fermentation results in foul-smelling faeces and wind. The food wastes pass through the large intestine (colon) where water is absorbed, resulting in a more solid mass travelling to the rectum before being passed as stool.

Changes in cystic fibrosis

As part of this process of moving nutrients from the inside of the gut into the bloodstream the cells lining the gut secrete fluid which aids lubrication and movement of the bolus through the intestine. In CF this secretion of intestinal fluid is impaired.

Pancreas

The pancreas is the gland in the abdomen which produces enzymes to digest foodstuffs (Figure 3.1). The enzymes are produced by cells in the pancreas and released into small channels which join together to form the pancreatic duct which in turn leads to the upper small intestine. As well as the enzymes (principally lipase, tryptase and amalyse) the pancreatic secretions are rich in bicarbonate and thus the enzymes are released in an alkaline soup into the small intestine. This bicarbonate-rich alkaline solution changes the pH of the intestinal contents from an acid environment on leaving the stomach to an alkaline environment in the small intestine.

In cystic fibrosis the small channels become blocked and decreased amounts of enzymes reach the small intestine. Humans have a large reserve of pancreatic

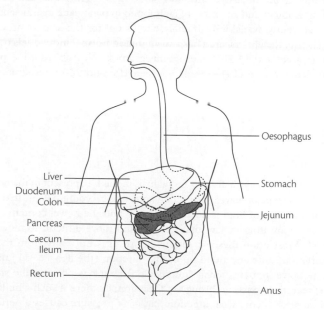

Figure 3.1 Diagram of the abdominal organs.

function so that less than 10 per cent of pancreatic function is required to provide enough enzymes for normal food digestion. Thus some individuals with cystic fibrosis are pancreatic-sufficient (i.e. have enough enzymes for digestion) but in the UK (and in the US) about 85 per cent of CF individuals are pancreatic-insufficient. Whether or not someone is pancreatic-sufficient is in part dependent on the combination of cystic fibrosis-causing mutations they have. It is important to remember that the pancreas is not normal even in pancreatic-sufficient CF individuals, and some people will become insufficient as they get older.

What happens to the pancreas in cystic fibrosis?

As the channels block, the cells producing enzymes stop functioning and eventually die and become scar tissue (fibrose). In pancreatic-sufficient individuals some cells die and others continue to function. Occasionally pancreatic-sufficient individuals can develop inflammation of the pancreas, known as pancreatitis, which gives abdominal pain. Cystic fibrosis sufferers with pancreatic insufficiency do not get pancreatitis.

How can you tell whether someone is pancreatic-insufficient?

Someone with pancreatic insufficiency generally has abnormal stools (fatty, slimy, frequent and offensive) and may fail to thrive. The stools can be examined for fat globules and an excess of fat is found in pancreatic insufficiency. The best test currently available is to analyse the stool for the level of an enzyme called elastase. Recent research has shown that in normal individuals the stool elastase is greater than 200 micrograms/gram stool, in borderline pancreatic sufficiency the stool elastase is between 100 and 200 micrograms/gram stool, and in individuals who are clearly insufficient stool elastase is less than 100 micrograms/gram stool.

Bowel

Meconium ileus

About 15 per cent of cystic fibrosis individuals in the UK present in the newborn period with the type of bowel obstruction known as meconium ileus. In the fetus intestinal secretion of fluid is decreased in CF and the bowel contents known as meconium are thus stickier than normal and more difficult to move along the bowel. Most often these secretions fail to pass normally from the small to the large intestine and build up at this junction (the ileo–caecal junction). The large bowel remains small (microcolon) as it has not had the stimulus of bowel secretions passing through it. Occasionally there is such a build-up of meconium at the ileo–caecal junction that back pressure causes a perforation of the small intestine while the infant is still in the womb. This can sometimes be picked up on abdominal x-rays after birth.

Management of meconium ileus

The infant with meconium ileus will present with vomiting and a distended abdomen. They will not have passed any meconium. An abdominal x-ray will confirm intestinal obstruction and may be suggestive of meconium ileus. If so then the infant may be treated with enemas containing gastrografin (a substance which shows on x-rays and which has detergent-like properties). In many cases this will clear the bowel. If the obstruction persists then a surgical operation is needed. At surgery an incision is made in the bowel and the meconium cleared out. Sometimes it is necessary to remove a piece of bowel and most often the bowel can be rejoined during that operation. However, if this is not possible then one end of the bowel is brought out to the surface of the skin to form a temporary ileostomy. The most common types of ileostomy are shown in Figure 3.2. The bowel is then rejoined a few weeks later after it has recovered fully.

Distal intestinal obstruction syndrome (DIOS)

In older children and adults with cystic fibrosis it is possible for the bowel contents to be sticky and move sluggishly through the bowel. This can be made worse by inadequate replacement enzymes. The child or adult will experience

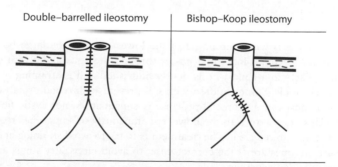

Figure 3.2 Ileostomy formation. (a) A double-lumen ileostomy. After a part of the bowel has been resected, both ends are brought to the skin surface to form an ileostomy. (b) The Bishop–Koop ileostomy. After a part of the bowel has been resected the bowel is rejoined in a T-formation with the leg of the T opening out on the skin as an ileostomy. As the bowel starts working stool content can go through to the lower bowel or pass out through the ileostomy.

abdominal pain which is sometimes, but not always, relieved by having the bowels open. Often the symptoms are picked up early at clinic reviews and sometimes the doctor can feel a soft mass in the lower right abdomen (at the ileo–caecal junction). Initial treatment at that early stage is to ensure adequate replacement enzymes and to ensure good fluid retention in the bowel by using medication such as lactulose or polyethylene glycol (Movicol). Sometimes DIOS can present acutely with abdominal pain, vomiting and failure to pass motions, i.e. acute or subacute bowel obstruction. Treatment then is in hospital with either oral treatments such as movicol or gastrografin or treatments using enemas. If the individual has had previous abdominal surgery it can be very difficult to distinguish acute or subacute obstruction due to DIOS, from obstruction due to adhesions.

Gastro-oesophageal reflux

Gastro-oesophageal reflux (GOR) is commoner in infants and children and probably also in adults with CF. Almost 20 per cent of infants less than 6 months old with CF have reflux compared with around 10 per cent of normal infants. Head-down positioning during physiotherapy may worsen GOR in infants and current advice is to avoid this position during physiotherapy in infancy. Recurrent reflux can worsen chest disease in some individuals and chest disease, resulting in over-inflation of the lungs can worsen reflux. Most GOR is managed with thickened feeds in infancy and acid-suppressing drugs. Only a small number of individuals with CF have GOR sufficiently severe to need surgical treatment.

Rectal prolapse

Rectal prolapse is when the lining of the lowest part of the large bowel – the rectum – becomes loose and passes through the anus along with stool. It is most likely in a child who is poorly nourished and is straining to pass large sticky stools. Some children with CF present with rectal prolapse but the commonest cause for rectal prolapse is constipation, not cystic fibrosis. The prolapse may return to the bowel spontaneously or sometimes requires gentle pressure to reduce it. The treatment is to try to avoid straining at stool, to ensure enzymes are at the correct dose, to avoid large fatty stools and to improve nutrition generally.

Intussusception

This is a rare condition where one portion of the intestine folds into the adjoining region (see Figure 3.3) and causes pain, blockage of the bowel and can also

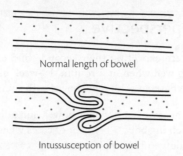

Normal length of bowel

Intussusception of bowel

Figure 3.3 Diagram of an intussusception. Note how the bowel has been pulled inside itself and become trapped.

damage the blood supply to the trapped portion of bowel. Intussusception can occur in normal children but is more common in cystic fibrosis. If the intussusception is in the large bowel then the inner portion of bowel can sometimes be pushed back by using an enema with air pressure. Treatment otherwise is surgical.

Bowel stricture

In the early 1990s there were an increasing number of reports of children with cystic fibrosis developing strictures in the large bowel, causing bowel obstruction and often requiring surgery. Investigations revealed two possible contributing factors:

1. A coating present in some types of replacement pancreatic enzymes – a methacrylic acid copolymer (Eudragit).

2. Very high amounts of enzymes being used.

Since the mid-1990s Eudragit has been removed from all replacement enzyme capsules and carers are advised to keep enzyme levels below 10,000 units of lipase per kilogram body weight per day for children. Bowel strictures are now very rarely seen.

Patient's perspective

John and Cathy were expecting their second child and the pregnancy seemed to be going well when at a routine 18-week ultrasound scan the infant was noted to have an echogenic bowel with some bowel dilatation.

There are many causes of echogenic bowel, including cystic fibrosis. Cystic fibrosis is seen in about 3 per cent of cases where there is no associated bowel dilatation and about 15 per cent of cases where the bowel is also dilated (European data).

The parents were given this information and both gave blood to test for the common CF gene mutations. Both parents were found to carry a single copy of *delta F508*. They were counselled that it was very likely the infant had cystic fibrosis and in view of the bowel dilatation that the infant might have bowel obstruction after birth (meconium ileus) and could require surgery. The obstetrician arranged for several further scans during the pregnancy and for the birth to be in a centre where neonatal surgery was provided.

Baby Joseph was born at term and intestinal obstruction confirmed. He had a gastrografin enema which showed a small under-used colon and nuggets of meconium in the large bowel, but dye did not pass into the small bowel. At surgery there was a very dilated section of bowel near the end of the small intestine which was excised and a double-barrelled ileostomy was brought to the skin. Joseph had an uneventful postoperative course, breastfed well and was discharged home at 7 days. He returned to hospital at 3 months of age and had his ileostomy closed.

4

How cystic fibrosis affects other organs

> ## ⮕ Key points
>
> ◆ Around 40 per cent of children with CF develop evidence of liver disease on testing but only in less than 5 per cent does it become severe enough to cause symptoms
>
> ◆ The likelihood of developing CF-related diabetes increases with age
>
> ◆ More than 25 per cent of adults with CF have diabetes
>
> ◆ Osteoporosis is common in adults with CF and more likely in those who are very thin, take little exercise and have chronic chest infection

Liver disease

The main function of the liver is to metabolize foodstuffs and drugs entering the bloodstream. The liver is another organ in the body which produces secretions (bile salts) that travel through small channels and in CF some of these channels (bile ducts) may become blocked, causing liver disease. Liver function can be assessed by measuring liver enzymes by a blood test and also by looking at the size and structure of the liver by an ultrasound scan. In early liver disease the liver enzymes can be raised and/or there can be abnormalities on liver ultrasound. The earliest ultrasound abnormality is an increase in the echogenicity or graininess of the liver picture indicating that there are patchy changes – likely reflecting blockage of some of the small channels. As liver disease progresses the ultrasound abnormalities become more obvious. Liver cirrhosis can develop with enlargement of the liver and back pressure on the flow of blood through the liver. This back pressure of blood can eventually cause enlargement of the spleen (another organ in the abdomen) and dilatation of blood vessels surrounding the bottom of the gullet (oesophageal varices).

Some abnormality of liver function is common and 40 per cent of children with cystic fibrosis develop evidence of liver involvement by the age of 10 years. However, it is uncommon for liver disease to be severe, and less than 5 per cent of cystic fibrosis individuals develop liver disease severe enough to cause symptoms (liver cirrhosis). If individuals reach adult life without liver disease they are unlikely to develop it.

What can be done if liver disease is detected early?

Cystic fibrosis patients will have some assessment of liver function each year – usually by blood test. Some CF units also do annual liver ultrasounds. This permits liver dysfunction to be picked up early. Ursodeoxycholic acid ('urso' for short) is a naturally occurring bile salt which has properties that help secretions move along the liver channels. There is good evidence that daily additional doses of Urso will result in a fall of raised liver enzymes. It is less clear whether its use affects the long-term development of severe liver disease.

Gallbladder disease

It is not uncommon for small gallstones to develop in CF. These are usually found incidentally at an annual review when an ultrasound scan of the liver and gallbladder is performed. Usually these stones cause no symptoms at all. Some doctors use the medicine Urso to try to dissolve the stones and some stones do disappear. Very occasionally a stone can get stuck in the passage from the gallbladder to the bowel and cause pain. This is known as cholecystitis.

Diabetes

Insulin is a hormone produced in the pancreas. Within the pancreas there are collections of cells known as islets of Langerhans. These are formed of beta cells, which produce insulin, and alpha cells, which produce another hormone – glucagon. Insulin is released directly into the bloodstream in response to glucose load. Insulin lowers the level of glucose in the blood by converting it to the carbohydrate glycogen, which is stored in the liver. In CF as the pancreas shrinks and becomes fibrotic some of the islet cells can be damaged and so less insulin is produced. Individuals with cystic fibrosis can then develop diabetes. This cystic fibrosis-related diabetes is different from the type 1 diabetes, which occurs in children and young adults where the body develops an autoimmune response to its own insulin-producing cells, and is also different to the type 2 diabetes which occurs in older and overweight adults.

Cystic fibrosis-related diabetes is unusual before the age of 10 years but 5 per cent of 11–17-year-olds, 12 per cent of 18–24-year-olds and more than 25 per cent of adults who are more than 25 years old develop diabetes. The development of CF diabetes is a gradual process: at first individuals are simply unable to produce enough insulin to handle a large glucose load and so have temporary high blood glucose after some meals or snacks (glucose intolerance). Gradually as insulin production fails the blood glucose remains high for more of the day. There have been studies showing that high blood glucose is related to more complications in cystic fibrosis, with more lung infection, decreased lung function and general ill-health before frank diabetes develops. For this reason all teenagers and young adults are tested for glucose intolerance on at least an annual basis, for example by oral glucose tolerance test or blood glucose checks after meals (postprandial). This early identification of people at risk of diabetes allows intervention to prevent a decline in lung function.

Treatment of diabetes

The goals in treating CF-related diabetes are to prevent negative effects of diabetes on nutrition and lung function as well as preventing long-term diabetic complications. Most people with CF diabetes need treatment with insulin by injection two to four times a day. They need to maintain a good high-energy diet with insulin doses adjusted to cope with this. Where possible complex carbohydrates such as bread, potatoes, pasta and cereals are preferred to sweets or sugary drinks. The diabetes can be controlled most easily if the same amount of food is eaten around the same time each day.

 Patient's perspective

James came for his annual review in February. He was 15 and had been diagnosed with CF at the age of 10 months when he was admitted to hospital with a bad chest infection. He felt he did not have much trouble from his CF and kept his chest clear with a mixture of physio, using an Acapella device with huffing and lots of football. He had noticed that although he was eating lots he did not seem to be putting on much weight. The whole family had a viral infection at Christmas time but James had noticed that he seemed to be taking longer than his brothers to regain his normal energy levels.

As part of his annual review James did a finger prick blood glucose test before breakfast (fasting) and five more tests 2 hours after main meals. The fasting blood glucose level was slightly above normal and four of the five levels after meals were high.

James was very upset to learn that he had CF-related diabetes and that he would need to have injections of insulin each day. However, he was prepared to learn more about it and was seen by the diabetic specialist and dietician. He was relieved that he would not have to make major changes to his diet and that he could still have his chocolate bar before football practice. He started with twice-daily injections and from the beginning did them himself. Within 2 months he had put on 3 kg in weight and was back in the football team with his usual level of energy.

He said, 'CF has always been part of life so I didn't mind too much about the treatment but I hate having diabetes. The injections and blood tests are a pain. I know if I miss them I'll feel rotten but it's hard to do every day without a break.'

Vitamin deficiencies

The vitamins A, D, E and K are fat soluble and therefore absorbed by the body along with fat. In CF fat, and therefore the fat-soluble vitamins, are poorly absorbed. Individuals with CF are routinely prescribed vitamin supplements but if they do not take them then over the years vitamin deficiencies can occur.

Vitamin A deficiency leads to abnormalities of vision particularly in poor light conditions (night blindness). Vitamin E deficiency can result in anaemia and in poor balance and muscle weakness. Vitamin D deficiency can result in osteoporosis and bones that fracture easily. Vitamin K deficiency can result in bruising or bleeding, particularly in individuals who also have liver disease.

Electrolyte abnormalities (pseudo Barter's syndrome)

This is an unusual condition caused by excessive salt (sodium) loss and usually occurs in infancy. The sodium may be lost in sweating but also by vomiting. The kidney then tries to compensate for the low body sodium by excreting other electrolytes such as potassium and hydrogen. The infant may be lethargic, sleepy, unable to feed, vomiting and generally unwell. A blood test reveals the abnormalities of electrolyte imbalance and treatment is with salt replacement.

Male infertility

Sperm normally pass from the testes first through a coiled tube called the epididymus, then through a small tube called the vas deferens. In CF the vas deferens becomes obstructed during fetal life and withers away. Most men with CF therefore produce sperm but the sperm cannot leave the testes, leading to infertility. Modern infertility management can provide solutions. (See Chapter 14.)

Clubbing

This is an abnormality of the nailbed where there is increased growth of tiny blood vessels which give the nailbed a softer or more fluctuant feeling on examination. As this progresses the angle between the nailbed and finger disappears. Eventually the whole fingertip may develop a rounded appearance. It is not really understood why this happens, but it can occur where there is chronic infection or inflammation in disorders such as CF or inflammatory bowel disease and also in conditions where there is poor oxygenation of the blood, for example in congenital heart disease.

Arthritis

Acute episodic arthritis occurs as an occasional complication of CF in teenage or early adult life. Arthritis seems to be more common in women. The individual will complain of joint pain, swelling and stiffness. The arthritis is sometimes accompanied by a rash. It usually responds to non-steroidal anti-inflammatory drugs such as ibruprofen. Occasional individuals need oral steroid treatment.

Osteoporosis

Throughout life bones have a continual cycle of growth, cell death and renewal. In recent years it has been recognized that most adults with CF make less new bone than normal and have thin bones which are more prone to fracture.

There may be many factors contributing to osteoporosis including suboptimal nutrition, poor absorption of calcium and vitamin D, steroids used in treatment, chronic infection and poor exercise capability. Fractures which are particularly difficult and important in cystic fibrosis are rib fractures and vertebral (backbone) fractures. Both of these make physiotherapy difficult and painful. Around one in three adults with CF has low bone density with women more frequently affected.

It is now recognized that preventative action needs to be taken during childhood as well as during adult life. It is important therefore for the bones as well as for general health to have good nutrition and take regular exercise. Calcium-rich foods such as dairy products and fish and regular supplementation of vitamin D are important during childhood in order to build up bone mass. Puberty seems to be a critical time. The thickness of bone (bone density) can be checked with a scan called a DEXA scan (which stands for dual energy x-ray absorptiometry). Normal values for bone density in childhood are not yet sufficiently consistent to be useful, but there are reliable normal values for adults and bone density should be checked throughout adult life. Treatment in those found to have low bone density involves attention to nutrition and exercise as above and in addition the use of a group of drugs called biphosphonates.

Incontinence of urine

Leakage of urine during coughing, physiotherapy or exercise is common in young women with cystic fibrosis. Until recently this was a hidden problem as women were embarrassed to talk about it. Surveys have shown that at least two-thirds of adult women with CF have some urinary leaks (compared with 5–10 per cent women without CF). Treatment is mainly by learning to improve muscle control with pelvic floor exercises and so a physiotherapist's help is essential.

5

Daily treatment for cystic fibrosis

➡ Key points

◆ People with CF should have a high-calorie, high-fat diet

◆ When supplementary enzymes are needed they should be taken with each meal and each snack

◆ Clearance of secretions from the lungs is improved with physiotherapy

◆ There are several different physiotherapy methods and a physiotherapy regimen should be adapted for each individual

◆ Monitoring for lung infection using cough swabs or sputum samples should be done at every clinic visit and for new symptoms of cough

◆ Early treatment of infection can prevent/control inflammation and lung damage

Daily treatment for the most young children with cystic fibrosis consists of enzymes taken with each meal or snack, once-daily vitamin supplements, twice-daily physiotherapy and antibiotics as indicated. These treatments are integrated around a normal life and the child is expected to be energetic, go to nursery or school, take part in all activities with other children and misbehave just as others do.

Nutrition

Diet

People with CF should have a normal diet. They are encouraged to aim for a diet that is high in calories and high in fat. The reason for this is that most CF individuals are pancreatic-insufficient. This means that they need supplementary enzymes to help digest their food. Supplementary enzymes are rarely as good as those produced naturally and so the recommendation is that someone with CF should aim to eat a diet which contains approximately 120 per cent of the normal calory requirements for a person of the same sex, weight and age but who does not have cystic fibrosis. The aim should be for 30–40 per cent of those calories to come from fat.

The CF care team recommends diets containing butter, milk, cheese and chocolate. There may be a conflict with 'healthy eating' campaigns promoted at school (see Chapter 10).

Pancreatic enzymes

For people with cystic fibrosis who are pancreatic-insufficient supplementary enzymes (enclosed in small capsules) are needed to help digest foodstuffs containing fat or protein and complex carbohydrates. Simple sugary sweets or fruits can be eaten without enzymes, but all other meals and snacks need enzymes taken alongside.

What is in the enzyme capsules?

Most commonly the capsules contain three enzymes: lipase, amylase and protease. Of these lipase, which helps break down fats, is the most important. The capsule coating dissolves in the stomach. This then releases granules which have a special coating on them which means that they are protected from the acid in the stomach, however the granules will then release the enzymes when they enter the alkaline environment of the upper small intestine.

How should enzyme capsules be taken?

It is best to swallow the capsules whole. Small children will not be able to achieve this so for them it is best to open the capsules and give them the contents on a spoon. For babies and other small children it is best to give the granules mixed with a little fruit purée such as apple on a teaspoon before they start a meal. They can also be given with yogurt on a spoon or breastfeeding mothers can express a little breast milk into which the granules may be mixed. It is important that the child does not crunch the granules as this releases the enzymes in the mouth and they are then inactive before they reach the small intestine. As soon as is possible the child should learn to swallow the capsules whole.

How many enzyme capsules should be taken?

The number of enzyme capsules required varies from person to person and depends on the amount of fat they are taking at any one snack or meal. As a rough rule of thumb 10,000 units of lipase should be taken with approximately 4.5 grams of fat. The British recommendation is that enzyme supplementation should not normally exceed 10,000 units of lipase per kilogram of body weight per day.

Enzyme capsules can come in different strengths and the strength is usually the number of units of lipase contained in that capsule – for example, Creon 10000, Creon 25000, Pancrease MT-10. It would be commonplace for a 7-year-old child weighting 24 kilograms to be taking 18 to 20 capsules of Creon 10 000 per day.

There are several brands of enzymes available and different ones in different countries, for example, Pancrease, Pancrease MS-8 and Ultrase MT-12, Ultrase MT-18, etc. There is also a preparation of granules with a small scoop such that there are 5000 units of lipase per scoop. As the different types all vary in what they contain and how they are made it is difficult to know the exact amount of active ingredients in the different enzymes and how many should be taken. In the USA in April 2004, a new rule was issued requiring makers of pancreatic enzyme supplements to get their drugs approved by the Food and Drug Administration (FDA) within the next four years. This will ensure that the manufacturing process of pancreatic enzymes is standardized, thus guaranteeing consistency of the capsules from batch to batch.

What if someone is taking high doses of enzymes but still has fatty stools or poor weight gain?

The pancreas normally produces enzymes in its secretions which are high in bicarbonate, i.e. the enzymes are in an alkaline soup. In pancreatic insufficiency there is decreased enzyme production and decreased alkaline material such that the upper small intestine may not be alkaline enough to permit the artificial enzyme granules to release the enzymes and work efficiently. To counter this it is sometimes necessary to decrease the amount of acid produced by the stomach by taking a medicine such as ranitidine or omeprazole.

Vitamins

Some vitamins, namely A, D, E and K, are fat soluble and absorbed into the body along with fats. In CF these vitamins are poorly absorbed and so higher doses than normally found in foods are needed. Vitamin supplements come as liquids for young children or as capsules. The recommended daily amounts are vitamin A 8000 IU, vitamin D 800 IU and vitamin E 200 IU (where IU stands for international units) but vitamin levels are generally checked at an annual review and doses adjusted as needed for the individual.

What would happen if vitamin supplements were not taken?

If vitamin levels become very low it can have an effect on a number of different areas of the body. For example in severe vitamin A deficiency individuals cannot see well in the dark, vitamin D is essential for good bone growth, vitamin E is essential to preserve the functioning of nerves in the body and vitamin K is involved in making sure that people do not bleed when they cut themselves. Some deficiencies can be corrected quickly by taking large doses of vitamins, for example vitamin K and vitamin A, but problems caused by deficiency in vitamins D and E take longer to remedy.

Physiotherapy

People with CF find it more difficult to clear normal secretions from the chest. Normally secretions are moved by the small hairs lining the airways (cilia), which waft the material from the small to the larger airways. Cough is a very effective way of clearing secretions from the larger airways. The aim of physiotherapy is to improve clearance of secretions to ensure air entry to all parts of the lungs. For most individuals with CF it is recommended that they have physiotherapy twice daily – in the mornings to clear any secretions that have collected overnight, and in the evenings before they go to bed.

The conventional physiotherapy technique is percussion and drainage and parents are taught how to perform this technique on infants and young children. As the child gets older other techniques are taught so that the child becomes independent of their parents for their physiotherapy.

Percussion and drainage

The child is placed in a position to favour emptying of one area of the lung and the chest is then clapped with a cupped hand at a rate of about three times per second. After about 2 minutes of clapping some deep breaths in with slow breaths out and then a huff or cough will clear any secretions. The child is then repositioned to tackle the next area of the lung.

Active cycle of breathing

The active cycle consists of breaths in and out using the lower chest followed by deep breaths in and slow breaths out then huffs to clear the airways (see below). The child can start to learn elements of this technique from age 5–6 years.

The active cycle of breathing

Active cycle of breathing is a technique which uses breathing exercises to:

♦ loosen and clear secretions

♦ improve ventilation.

Active cycle of breathing can be performed in sitting, lying or postural drainage positions.

Active cycle of breathing uses an alternating depth of breathing to move phlegm from the small airways at the bottom of your lungs to larger airways near the top where it can be cleared more easily with huffing/coughing.

The parts of the active cycle of breathing are:

Breathing control This is normal gentle breathing using the lower chest, with relaxation of the upper chest and shoulders. It helps you to relax between the deep breathing and huffing.

Deep breathing These are slow deep breaths in followed by relaxed breaths out. Three to four deep breaths are enough.

Huffing This is a medium-sized breath in, followed by a fast breath out through an open mouth, using the muscles of the chest and stomach to force the breath out. This will move secretions along the airways to a point where you can cough them up.

Coughing This should follow two to three huffs or a deep breath in. Don't cough unless secretions are ready to be cleared.

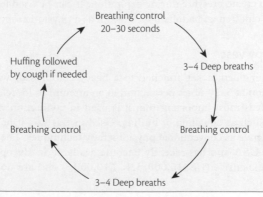

41

Autogenic drainage

This technique consists of a three-phase breathing regimen designed to move secretions from the very small airways to the larger major airways. It avoids forceful breathing out. In general this technique is more difficult to learn and is most successful in adolescents and adults. It is widely used in Europe.

PEP systems

These are devices to help with physiotherapy. The PEP (positive expiratory pressure) mask is a face mask which delivers a positive pressure while breathing out. The pressure is set individually for a patient. A similar device can be used with a mouthpiece rather than a mask. It may open up airways that are otherwise blocked and by widening the airway allow air behind mucus and then help move the mucus in conjunction with a forced breath out or huff.

Flutter

In the flutter a steel ball vibrates against a cone causing air-flow vibration (Figure 5.1). This causes a vibratory pressure when breathing through it. It is thought that the vibration in the airways can mobilize secretions. The flutter has to be carefully positioned at an angle and is gravity-dependent, that is, it cannot be used when lying down.

Acapella

The Acapella is a device which combines both PEP and vibration. There is a counterweighted plug and magnet to create the vibration and an adjustable valve to create pressure during expiration. It can be used in any position. Many older children and adults find it useful as a physiotherapy aid.

The therapy vest

This is an air-filled jacket attached to a heavy compressor which provides chest vibration at 5–20 times per second in an attempt to loosen and mobilize secretions. It is most important that it is used in conjuction with clearance techniques such as coughing or huffing. Used in this way it has been shown to be as effective as conventional physiotherapy techniques. The vest is widely used in the USA and has recently become available in Europe. The devices are very expensive (US\$16,000; UK £10,000+) and are not available on the NHS.

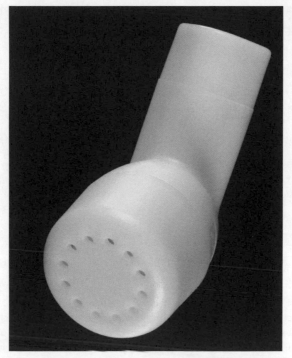

Figure 5.1 A flutter device. The individual breathes out slowly through this pipe-like device. Inside the pipe the 'ball-bearing' moves up and down creating a vibratory sensation which is transmitted back to the airways.

Exercise

Exercise has a very important role in keeping the lungs clear of mucus secretions. It encourages deep breathing and can be a very enjoyable part of treatment (and life) for many children. Bouncing games and trampolining are very useful physiotherapy aids. Exercise should be a supplement to and not a substitute for physiotherapy.

Short-term studies of exercise programmes in cystic fibrosis have shown benefits including:

- decreased breathlessness

- increased sputum clearance

- increased cardiorespiratory fitness

- improved morale and quality of life.

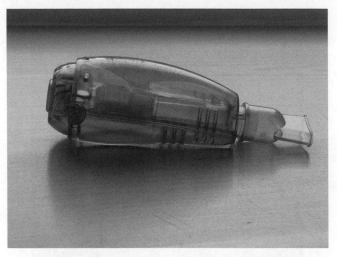

Figure 5.2 An Acapella. This device combines an expiratory resistance with a vibratory pressure.

A mixture of exercise types is useful. For example endurance exercises might include swimming, running, cycling, trampolining or skipping. Strength exercises such as sprint training or in older children and adults weight training are useful. Exercise should be sufficiently frequent and intense enough to improve cardiorespiratory fitness. A general recommendation would be 20–30 minutes three to four times a week.

Generally children enjoy exercise but the vigorous resistance type of training can cause a repetitive stress on growing bones and joints. It is important therefore to have a varied programme rather than to concentrate on one type of exercise only.

 FAQ

Why should I do physiotherapy when I/my child is well?

It is difficult to maintain the discipline of twice-daily physiotherapy in a busy life if there is no immediate benefit, e.g. no cough or sputum produced. However, it is an important preventative technique to ensure that secretions do not quietly accumulate in the lungs and block the smallest airways. It should be regarded very much the same as cleaning teeth twice daily. If physiotherapy becomes part of the daily routine it is much easier for the child to accept physiotherapy when they are unwell. It is, however, very difficult to prove whether physiotherapy is useful in a child without symptoms, but some studies underway are attempting to test this.

Which physiotherapy technique is best?

There have been some studies looking at the different techniques and examining whether, for example, the therapy vest is better than percussion and drainage or whether exercise alone is as good. Overall they show that no one technique is better than the others but all physiotherapy techniques are better than exercise alone.

Making physio fun

It is useful to try to make physiotherapy time a special individual time for parent and child together rather than a daily chore. Using blowing games, for example bubbles, noisy blowing toys, incorporating play – the child as wheelbarrow for chest drainage – tickling and laughing to encourage deep breaths and coughs, and using favourite videos or storytelling can make physio time special.

Julie said: 'Evie's physio is going really well. I never thought it would get to this stage. It was so difficult at the beginning but it's part of everyday life now and she even reminds me if I forget.'

Antibiotics

CF patients find it difficult to clear infection from their lungs. An important part of treatment therefore is monitoring for infection by using either cough swabs or sputum samples and treating any infection which is found.

In young children one of the commonest bugs (bacteria) which can cause infection is called *Staphylcoccus aureus* (known as *Staph.* for short). It is usual in the UK (but not in the USA) for newly diagnosed infants to be put on an anti-*Staphylococcus* antibiotic in a preventative way for the first year or two of their life. The most common antibiotic used in this way in called flucloxacillin.

When it is taken as a preventative antibiotic it is used only twice daily. For treatment of diagnosed infections, flucloxacillin is used four times a day.

On each visit to a cystic fibrosis clinic or if a new cough develops individuals will have either a cough swab or sputum sample taken and tested for bacteria. Any bacteria found will be treated. Most commonly this is with oral antibiotics, however there are some bacteria, such as *Pseudomonas aeruginosa*, which respond poorly to oral treatment alone. Inhaled antibiotics delivered by means of a nebulizer are often used for treatment of *Pseudomonas aeruginosa*, often in combination with the oral antibiotic ciprofloxacin. (See Chapter 8 for further information on micro-organisms.)

Long-term antibiotics

As well as the preventative use of flucloxacillin there are other indications for the long-term use of antibiotics. Some people have recurrent growths of the same bacteria and they often benefit from using a specific antibiotic on a daily basis, sometimes for many years. This does not cause long-term problems with immunity. In addition a specific oral antibiotic called azithromycin also appears to have anti-inflammatory properties and in particular has been shown to improve lung function in those patients chronically infected with *Pseudomonas aeruginosa* when used either on a daily or a three times a week basis.

Inhaled antibiotics

There are currently two common inhaled antibiotics available. The first, colomycin, has been used for many years in Europe and the UK. It can suppress and kill *Pseudomonas aeruginosa* and in individuals who are chronically infected it can control the infection for many years. It is generally given once or twice daily over several months and can be used for many years. The other, called Tobi, a commercially available variety of the antibiotic tobramycin, is newer and is used very widely in the USA as well as in Europe and the UK. It is generally used on a one-month-on, one-month-off system. Some individuals who find they have more symptoms on their month off will use colomycin and Tobi on alternate months. Some other antibiotics such as gentamicin can also be used in a nebulizer.

Intravenous antibiotics

Antibiotics are used intravenously if the child/adult is unwell with an infection or if the infection is caused by a bacterium poorly sensitive to oral drugs. Usually these are initially given in hospital, but many families are taught how to give intravenous antibiotics and complete the course at home. There are home-care companies who will deliver intravenous antibiotics ready made up so giving at home is made easier.

Portacath

A portacath is a small device placed beneath the skin which allows direct access to a major blood vessel (Figures 5.3 and 2.5c). It is very useful for individuals who have to have repeated courses of intravenous antibiotics.

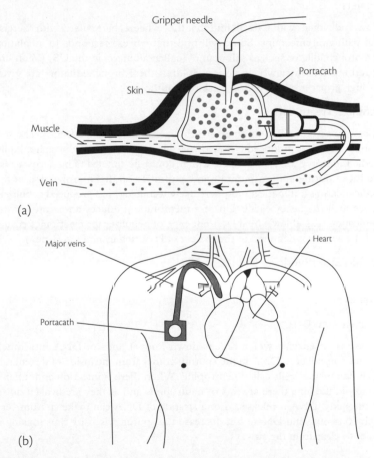

Figure 5.3 Diagram of a portacath. (a) The portacath lies under the skin and is accessed by a needle when needed. A small tube leads directly into a major blood vessel. (b) Position of a portacath.

When access is needed a small needle is placed through the skin into the portacath and the needle left in place till the course of antibiotics is finished when it is removed. Between courses a needle is placed into the portacath once a month and the device flushed to keep it clear.

Additional forms of treatment

Respiratory

Inhalers

Many individuals with CF will find that they wheeze, particularly with exercise and with viral infections. Some will find that wheeze responds to inhalation of a bronchodilator such as salbutamol (called albuterol in the US) (Ventolin) or terbutaline (Bricanyl). In young children these bronchodilators are given through a spacer device with a mask or mouthpiece.

Nebulizer treatments

There are several different types of nebulizer available (Figure 5.4). The traditional nebulizer produced a flow of gas which when driven through a liquid medication produced an aerosol which could be inhaled. The aerosol was produced during both inspiration and expiration so that a proportion of the medication was lost to the atmosphere. New technology has produced nebulizers where high-frequency oscillation of a membrane produces an aerosol of the medication (e.g. eFlow). In at least one type of nebulizer the electronics ensure that the aerosol is delivered to the patient only during inspiration (I-neb).

Nebulized antibiotics

As detailed above, some individuals use long-term antibiotics delivered by nebulizer.

Dornase alfa (DNase)

DNase is an enzyme which breaks down long strands of DNA into much shorter components. DNA in the sputum comes from the inside of degenerating inflammatory cells called neutrophils. When there is infection and inflammation in the lung there are lots of neutrophils and as they are broken down by the body, DNA is released. Long strands of DNA can make sputum very sticky (viscous) and DNase can decrease the sputum viscosity thus making it easier to clear from the airways.

DNase is inhaled using a nebulizer once daily. It is generally used in individuals who have difficulty clearing mucus from the airways and have decreased lung function. It should be used either after physiotherapy or at least 45 minutes

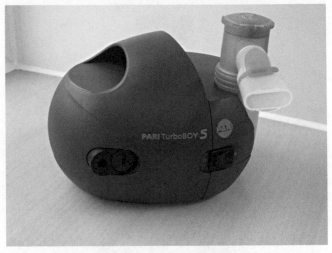

(a)

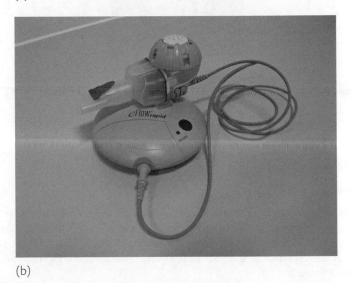

(b)

Figure 5.4 Three types of nebulizer: (a) PARI; (b) eFlow (continues overpage).

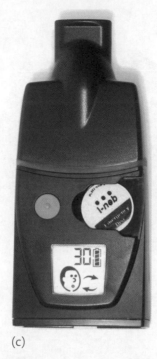

(c)

Figure 5.4 *(continued)*. (C) I-neb.

before physiotherapy takes place. It is an expensive drug and not every individual benefits from it: however, if it is shown to improve lung function then it should be continued long-term.

Hypertonic saline

Strong concentrations of saline (hypertonic) delivered by nebulizer have also been shown to clear mucus from the airways in some people with cystic fibrosis. In some studies the effects have been as good as DNase. It seems that some individuals respond well to hypertonic saline, some do not respond and some cannot tolerate it.

Oxygen

There may be times during an acute severe infection when the lungs cannot deliver enough oxygen to the bloodstream and short-term supplementary oxygen may be needed. This is generally given in hospital.

As lung disease in cystic fibrosis progresses the lungs may become less able to maintain oxygen levels, particularly at night time or during exercise. For these individuals with severe disease oxygen can be provided at home and portable oxygen for exercise.

Nutritional

Food supplements

Some people with CF find it difficult to eat enough to meet their energy needs. High-calorie food supplements are available. Many of these are milk-based or are added to milk, e.g. Scandishake, but high-calorie carbohydrate drinks are also available. Complex carbohydrates can also been added to infant feeds, e.g. Maxijul. A dietician can supply ideas and recipes for using these food substances in drinks, cakes and meals.

Overnight feeds

For some people, despite their best efforts, it can be difficult to maintain a sufficiently high energy intake. During adolescence, for example, very high calorie intake is needed to ensure optimal growth. If growth is faltering then overnight feeds may be considered. Overnight feeds are given either through a tube passing through the nose into the stomach (nasogastric tube) or via a small tube passing directly from the skin into the stomach (a gastrostomy) and are slowly dripped into the stomach over 6–8 hours. Weight gain can be very impressive after overnight feeds are started (see Figure 5.5).

Ursodeoxycholic acid

This is a naturally occurring bile salt which has properties that stimulate the flow of bile through the small channels in the liver. Extra ursodeoxycholic acid is given to individuals who show evidence of liver disease.

Management of care

Cystic fibrosis is a complex, chronic disorder and is best looked after by a multi-disciplinary team. CF centres have been established around the UK, Europe, North America and many other countries and are responsible for directing the care for the patients in their area. There is good evidence that individuals with CF do better when their care is directed through a CF centre. Many paediatric CF centres will share care of their patients with paediatricians in local district general hospitals. Most adult CF centres provide all the care for their patients. In general a CF centre will have two or more paediatricians/physicians with a major interest in CF who will work with a team consisting of CF nurse specialists,

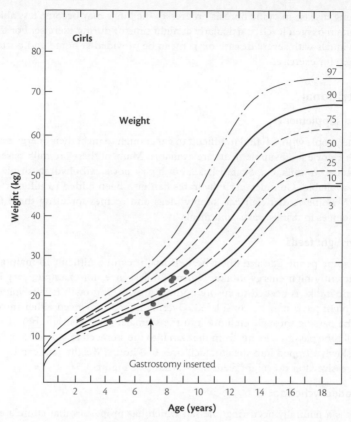

Figure 5.5 Weight chart showing impressive weight gain after overnight feeding was started.

physiotherapists, dieticians, psychologists, social workers and pharmacists, all of whom will have expertise in cystic fibrosis. These specially trained individuals will be available to help people with cystic fibrosis and their families as they are needed.

The clinic visit

When someone is newly diagnosed with cystic fibrosis they will be seen very regularly in clinic to make sure that they are managing their treatment. Once things are settled clinic appointments occur regularly every 2 to 3 months. At each visit the patient will be seen by the CF nurse and doctor, is likely also to see the physiotherapist and dietician, and others such as the psychologist may be seen by arrangement. Height and weight will be checked, a cough swab or sputum specimen will be taken and sent for culture, and if the patient is old enough to manage the technique then simple lung function tests will be performed.

Annual review

The CF centre will perform an annual review on each patient. This is to assess how well the patient has done during the year and to pick up any early abnormalities which may indicate that a change of treatment is necessary. The way an annual review is performed will differ between centres: in some parts of the country the entire CF team will travel to a local district general hospital and in others the patient will travel to the CF centre. Common elements in the annual review will be:

◆ blood tests

◆ chest x-ray

◆ sputum/cough swab

◆ dietary assessment

◆ physiotherapy assessment

◆ lung function assessment

◆ clinical examination

and may also include ultrasound examination of liver, lung scans and exercise tests.

At the end of the review when all the results are available they will be discussed with the patient and their families and summaries sent to the local paediatrician and to the family doctor.

Hospital admissions

Most care for CF patients takes place at home and so admissions to hospital have become less common. However, at times of severe infection when intravenous drug therapy is required along with concentrated physiotherapy or oxygen therapy, hospital admission is essential. Hospital admissions are also needed at times of CF complications, such as distal intestinal obstruction syndrome (DIOS), intussusception or pneumothorax. Hospital admission may also be in order to perform an elective surgical procedure such as the insertion of a portacath or a gastrostomy.

Costs of care

Cystic fibrosis is expensive. There are costs in clinic and hospital visits as well as costs of drugs and equipment (see Table 5.1 for drug costs). In the UK the costs are met by the National Health Service but drugs are carefully prescribed to ensure they are used only where there is evidence of benefit. In Europe access to therapies is partially dependent on the state health services and partly on individual health insurances. In the USA health is funded by private insurance and by the state for those without insurance (Medicaid). Data from the Cystic Fibrosis Foundation shows that roughly 60 per cent of CF children in the USA are covered by private insurance schemes and 40 per cent depend on state care. The Cystic Fibrosis Foundation established a specialty pharmacy (Cystic Fibrosis Services Inc.) in 1988 to provide availability and access to CF medications as well as assistance with the complex insurance issues faced in obtaining these medications.

UK benefits: disability living allowance

It is recognized that cystic fibrosis is a chronic disease and that it is costly to look after someone with CF. Children need increased care and time from parents or carers; when grown up they need to spend additional time on their own treatment. For these reasons, in the UK, CF patients (or their parents to age 16 years) are entitled to claim a non-means-tested allowance called disability living allowance (DLA). This is paid at three different levels which should depend on how much additional care the individual needs. Unfortunately there is much variation across the UK in how CF individuals are graded for DLA.

Table 5.1 US prices taken from CF Services 2007. UK prices taken from British National Formulary 2007

Medication	Quantity	Price US	Price UK
Acid reducers			
Omeprazole 20 mg caps	30	$109.60	£12.60
Ranitidine 150 mg tabs	60	$80.81	£1.30
Ranitidine syrup (480 ml)	1	$323.84	£33.21
Antibiotics (oral)			
Ciprofloxacin 500 mg tabs	100	$525.80	£17.10
Azithromycin 200 mg tabs	30	$250.05	£67.15
Enzymes			
Creon 10000	100	$91.28	£16.66
Pancrease MT-10 caps	100	$105.26	–
Nebulized medication			
Colomycin	2 million unit vial	$50.16	£3.09
Dornase alfa (Pulmozyme-DNase)	30 ampoules	$1,641.75	£555.60
Tobi	56 ampoules	$3,465.59	£1,484.00
Nutritional supplements			
Duocal (14 oz can)	1	$24.08	£13.13
Scandishake	36	$61.92	£68.40
Vitamins			
ADEK paediatric drops (60 ml bottle)	1	$9.99	–
Vitamin E (400 IU caps)	100	$10.00	£17.23
Dalavit multivitamins	50 ml	–	£4.85
Vitamin A and D capsules	20	–	£0.64

Patient's perspective

'A Day in the Life of Me' by Macauley, aged 11 years

I have to get up really early so that I have time to do my physio before I go to school. It takes half an hour; my dad does it for me, whilst I watch telly. Before I start my physio I have an inhaler and then I have another one when I've finished. When that's finished I have a nebulizer called colomycin which takes about ten minutes.

After that I can get ready for school and have my breakfast.

When I have my breakfast I have to take lots of tablets. I have two types of vitamins, a hay-fever tablet, a tablet called Losec, an antibiotic and then Creon. I have to take lots of Creon everyday. Every time I eat I need Creon.

Then I get my school bag ready making sure that I remember my tablets.

Then my Mum takes me to school.

When I get home from school, I have another session of physio if I need it, and then my inhalers and another nebulizer called DNase.

Then I play, and play and play!

When I have my tea I have to have more Creon and also a different antibiotic.

Then, the worst bit of my day – homework!

Then I'll play or watch telly, then bed.

My day is pretty much the same as everyone's, it's just that I have to take tablets and have physio. It's all just part of our family life.

Patient's perspective

Jessica was always an active child. At the age of 4 years her parents bought a large trampoline for the garden and she spent many happy hours on it. Her mother then discovered that there were trampoline classes at a local leisure centre and Jessica started going every week from age 7 as a junior. She started training competitively and enjoyed learning the set routines. Last year she was second in the regional final. Her CF has not held her back.

6

The cystic fibrosis team

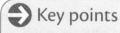 Key points

- All individuals with CF should have their care managed through a cystic fibrosis centre

- The cystic fibrosis team consists of doctors, nurses and therapists who have been specially trained in CF care and see large numbers of children and adults with CF

Cystic fibrosis is ideally managed at a CF specialist centre. If individuals live close to a centre all their care will be given there, but if they live further afield then care may be shared between the CF centre and their local hospital.

At the CF centre the team will consist of:

- Senior doctors (consultants) with special training and experience in CF who spend a substantial part of their working week looking after patients with CF.

- Junior doctors part way through their training in CF.

- CF nurse – the single most important person for families. They generally spend their time exclusively in CF care and will get to know families well. They will make home visits as well as seeing patients in outpatients and when in hospital and are the most important coordinating person. They are the first point of call for individuals with CF and provide support, advice and education as well as practical care.

♦ CF physiotherapist. The physiotherapist sees individuals at every visit and makes an assessment of the amount of mucus in the airways (bronchial secretions). Techniques of airway clearance are taught which are relevant to the age of the child and the extent of their lung disease. Advice on fitness and exercise regimens is provided.

♦ CF dietician. The dietician will monitor growth and nutritional status and see individuals regularly. The dietician will help with adjusting enzyme therapy, give advice on infant feeds, weaning, managing feeding behavioural problems and using food supplements if needed. They are critically involved in decision-making about overnight feeds and management of complications such as diabetes.

♦ CF social worker. The social worker is available as needed to support individuals and families. They may be able to give advice on school and employment issues and the patient's rights to allowances to ease financial difficulties.

♦ CF psychologist. It is important to have a psychologist available to see all families. There are invariably issues that occur as families and then individuals come to terms with a chronic disease. The CF psychologist has good knowledge of the disease and its treatments as well as the common problems that occur.

♦ Secretary/data manager. It is essential that there is good office back-up. There needs to be good communication with the patient's local hospital and with their family doctor as well as the patient themselves. In addition the organization of outpatient visits and annual reviews is complicated and time-consuming in large centres.

♦ Laboratory services:

– Bacteriology laboratories – for analysis of cough/sputum swabs.

– Lung function laboratories – for lung function tests.

– Radiology services – for chest radiographs (x-rays) and scans.

– Biochemical/haematology/immunology laboratories – to analyse all the blood samples.

– Genetics – for counselling of families and access to genetic testing as needed.

The local hospital will also have doctors and therapists with a special interest in CF but they will spend much of their time with other patients. There is generally excellent communication between the specialist centre and the local team by phone, email or letter and in many places there will be visits to the local hospital by members of the specialist centre team.

7
Nutrition in cystic fibrosis

> **⟶ Key points**
>
> ◆ Children with CF on a high-calorie, high-fat diet should grow normally
>
> ◆ At times of illness or during periods of fast growth, for example adolescence, high-calorie food supplements may be helpful
>
> ◆ A huge variety of food supplements is available
>
> ◆ Occasionally additional calories are needed and liquid supplements can be given slowly overnight into the stomach through either a nasogastric tube or a gastrostomy

There has been good evidence since the 1970s that a high-fat, high-calorie diet leads to a normal growth pattern and improved survival in cystic fibrosis. The aim therefore is that children with CF should grow normally and achieve a normal adult height and weight. In the majority of CF patients a high-calorie diet with adequate pancreatic supplementation achieves this, but for some nutrition remains a problem.

Poor nutrition in CF may result from a combination of factors including increased loss of fat (calories) in the stool; decreased appetite when feeling unwell and hence poor intake; or increased energy needs particularly during infection.

Growth surveillance and dietary advice are an important part of management. Each child will have their height and weight checked at each clinic visit. An individual's weight should be appropriate for their height. Growth charts for age based on large numbers of normal children are available (growth centile charts). A percentage weight for height can be calculated from the growth charts (normal greater than 85 per cent). Another simple assessment is to calculate the body mass index.

Body mass index (BMI) is the weight (in kg) divided by height squared (in m). The normal BMI varies throughout childhood and has to be related once again to a normal centile chart. The BMI is stable once final height is achieved and adults should have a BMI greater than 19.

In childhood dietary intervention would be considered if the child's weight for height was less than 85 per cent or if they had weight loss or a plateau in weight over two clinic visits (4–6 months). Similarly adults with a BMI of less than 19 or loss of weight over a few months would be targeted.

A dietician is involved from diagnosis and as neonatal screening becomes universal preventative counselling may decrease future nutritional problems.

Feeding the newborn baby

Normal growth rates can be achieved in infants with CF whether they are breastfed or bottle-fed. Breastfeeding has advantages for infants with cystic fibrosis as for other infants. In addition the enzyme content of breast milk may partially compensate for decreased pancreatic secretion in the infant, and it may offer some increased protection against infection. There is no evidence that any one brand of formula milk is superior to another. Dietary fat provides approximately 50 per cent of the energy intake of infants. Pancreatic enzyme replacement therapy should be introduced once there is evidence of malabsorption. The stools may be examined directly for fat globules and pancreatic insufficiency confirmed by measurement of faecal elastase. In the UK over 85 per cent of infants with CF are pancreatic-insufficient by 1 year of age.

Pancreatic enzymes should be given on a teaspoon mixed with a little fruit purée near the beginning or at intervals throughout the feed. The initial starting dose is usually a quarter to half a capsule (2500–5000 IU lipase) per milk feed and the dose is then adjusted for an individual infant.

Weaning can proceed as normal but some high-energy foods such as butter and cheese should be incorporated in the weaning diet.

Toddlers

Eating habits are developed at this age and advice from a dietician can be very useful, as all children will have some behavioural issues over foods at this age.

Parents may find this very difficult when there is also a feeling of pressure over ensuring the energy intake is high. It is important that parents feel confident in their long-term strategy and relaxed when there is normal day-to-day variation in intake so that long-term behavioural issues over food do not develop.

Childhood and adolescence

A normal diet with lots of high-energy foods is required. Occasionally high-energy food supplements may be used – particularly at times of illness. Normal adolescence is a time of peak growth and the dietary requirements are very high and additionally so in CF. Some young people find it difficult to maintain intake during this time and compliance with treatment regimens including pancreatic enzymes can be haphazard during adolescence. Regular food supplements can be very helpful.

Oral food supplements

If weight gain is poor despite dietary manipulation additional nutritional supplements can be used to complement the normal diet. It is best if they are taken after a meal or as an interim snack so they do not depress appetite. Supplements can be carbohydrate-only and added to drinks, e.g. Maxijul or Polycal. They can be stand-alone supplements available as juices ready to drink, e.g. Fresubin or Fortisip or they can be supplements available to mix with milk, e.g. Scandishake. Many flavours are available and it is usually necessary to provide the child with a selection so that they can choose those they like the most.

Table 7.1 Commonly used supplements (C is carbohydrate, F is fat, P is protein)

Supplement	Content	How taken	Calorie content
Maxijul	C	Add to drinks	2–4 kcal/g
Duocal	F and C	Add to drinks	5 kcal/g
Calogen	F	Drink or add to drink	4.5 kcal/mL
Scandishake	P, F and C	Mix with milk	2.5 kcal/mL
Emsogen	F	Dilute/add to drinks	0.8 kcal/mL*
Enlive (Ensure plus juice)	P and C	Ready to drink	1.5 kcal/mL

(continued)

Table 7.1 Commonly used supplements *(continued)*

Supplement	Content	How taken	Calorie content
Ensure Plus	P, F and C	Ready to drink	1.5 kcal/ml
Fortisip	P, F and C	Ready to drink	1.5 kcal/ml
Fortifresh	P, F and C	Yogurt	1.5 kcal/ml
Fortijuce	P, C	Drink	1.5 kcal/ml
Fresubin	P, F and C	Ready to drink	1 kcal/ml
Liquigen	F	Drink or add to drink	4.5 kcal/ml
Resource	P, F and C	Ready to drink	2 kcal/ml
ProCal Shot	P and F	Drink	4.5 kcal/ml

*At a 1 in 5 dilation..

Overnight feeds

Some individuals simply cannot eat enough food plus supplements during the day to meet their needs. Additional supplements can be given overnight using either feeding through a nasogastric tube or by placing a gastrostomy, a small tube passing through the skin directly into the stomach (Figure 7.1).

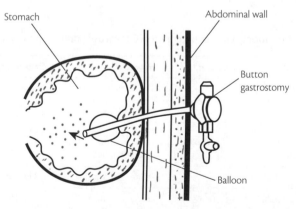

Figure 7.1 Diagram of a gastrostomy. The outside can be closed when not in use. The gastrostomy leads directly into the stomach with a balloon in the inside preventing it becoming dislodged.

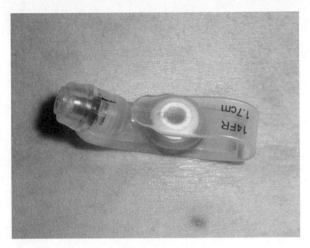

Figure 7.2 Photograph of a button gastrostomy.

Nasogastric tubes are simple and are most often used for short-term support during a period of illness in hospital, for example with a chest infection. A well-motivated mature individual can learn to pass them each night at home but for long-term feeding most people opt for a gastrostomy. The gastrostomy is usually sited under general anaesthetic and has a 'button' to close it off during the day (Figure 7.2). Over a period of several hours during sleep feed is slowly pumped through the gastrostomy into the stomach. An additional 1000–1500 calories per day can be achieved in this way. Many feeds require additional pancreatic enzymes and most conveniently these are taken at the beginning and middle or end of a feed. However, there are some feeds which provide fat and protein in partly broken-down forms (elemental) which can be used without additional pancreatic enzymes.

8

Micro-organisms in the cystic fibrosis lung

→ Key points

◆ *Staphylococcus aureus* is the bacteria most commonly found in young children with CF and is treated with an oral antibiotic

◆ *Pseudomonas aeruginosa (P. aeruginosa)* is a bacteria which occurs naturally in warm moist environments and is particularly attracted to the lung in CF

◆ Early treatment of *P. aeruginosa* infection with oral plus inhaled or intravenous antibiotics can usually prevent chronic infection

◆ Hygiene measures are important to prevent cross-infection between patients with CF

At every clinic visit and whenever there is a change in chest symptoms a sample should be taken to look for infection with bugs (bacteria). In young children and older people who cannot produce any sputum a cough swab is done. The child is asked to open their mouth widely and a swab is held at the back of the throat while they are asked to cough. Babies cannot cough to order and the cough swab stimulates a cough by tickling the back wall of the throat. There can be times when repeated cough samples are negative but there is nevertheless concern that there is infection in the lung. In these cases an investigation called bronchoscopy with bronchoalveolar lavage is performed.

A bronchoscopy can be performed either under a general anaesthetic or with deep sedation. A small flexible tube with a camera on the end is passed through the nose and voicebox into the airways. The airways can be seen and the amount of secretions and inflammation can be estimated. A very small area of the lung is then washed out and the secretions collected – this is what is meant by a lavage. These secretions can be cultured for micro-organisms and a sample also examined to assess the amount of inflammation present.

Bacteria found in the CF lung

Staphylococcus aureus

In young children with cystic fibrosis a bacterium called *Staphylococcus aureus* is a common lung invader. For this reason in the UK and in much of Europe (but not in the USA) young children are treated prophylactically with an anti-Staphylococcal antibiotic for the first year or two of life. There is some evidence that this decreases the amount of infection with *S. aureus*. Some individuals have recurrent isolations of *S. aureus* despite treatment and are on anti-Staphylococcal antibiotics continuously for many years.

Other common bacteria

Other common bacteria are *Haemophilus influenzae* and *Moraxella catarrhalis*. These are generally easily treated with oral antibiotics but in some individuals may return many times and again a continuous antibiotic may be indicated. These bacteria are common following a viral upper respiratory tract infection. *Streptococcus pneumoniae* infection can occur in cystic fibrosis but seems little commoner than in the normal population.

Pseudomonas aeruginosa

Pseudomonas aeruginosa is found in many natural environments. It thrives in warm moist environments and can be found where there is organic material and in soil and water. Everyone comes in contact with *Pseudomonas aeruginosa* (*P. aeruginosa*) and up to 10 per cent of healthy individuals may excrete it from their gut at any one time.

There have been several studies looking at how common and how early *P. aeruginosa* infection appears in children with CF. By one year of age between 19 and 33 per cent of children and by the age of 2 years up to 49 per cent of children will have had at least one isolation of *P. aeruginosa* on cough/throat swab. It is likely that some isolations found on cough/throat swab are infection of the upper respiratory tract only and do not involve the lower airways. There have been studies comparing simultaneous isolations from cough swab with samples taken directly from a lavage of a segment of the lower airways (done using bronchoscopy and bronchoalveolar lavage). Where there was a negative cough swab it was very unlikely that there was *P. aeruginosa*

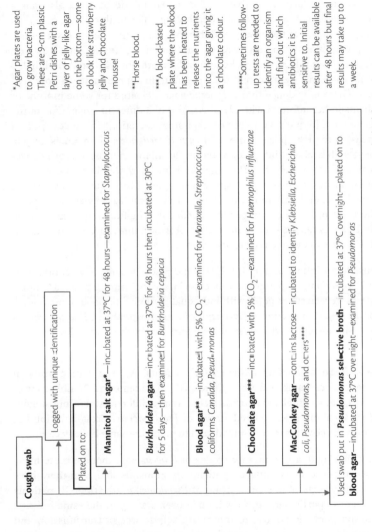

Figure 8.1 What happens to a cough swab/sputum sample. The journey through the laboratory.

found in the lower airways but a positive swab did not always correlate with *P. aeruginosa* from the lower airways.

In recent years it has become clear that the environment in the cystic fibrosis lung is particularly attractive to *P. aeruginosa*. The bacteria also has a number of defences which it can employ against antibiotics, e.g. it can settle on the surface of the airway and then produce a mucous coat surrounding and protecting it from lung defences and antibiotics (a biofilm). However, if the *P. aeruginosa* infection is picked up early treatment with oral and inhaled antibiotics can usually eradicate it from the lung (in approximately 85 per cent of cases). There is evidence that if *P. aeruginosa* is cleared for some months or years then another infection with *P. aeruginosa* is of a different strain. One of the main benefits of frequent sampling of respiratory secretions (cough or sputum specimens) is to pick up early infection with *P. aeruginosa*. Sometimes despite treatment with oral and inhaled antibiotics for many months and/or intravenous antibiotic treatment the *P. aeruginosa* is not completely eradicated and can be found in cough swabs or sputum samples. This is known as chronic infection. In general children and adults with chronic *Pseudomonas* infection have more symptoms and a more rapid decline in lung function. However, the organism can usually be kept under control with continuous use of inhaled antibiotics, either colomycin or tobramycin.

It is sensible for individuals with CF to avoid places where heavy contamination of *P. aeruginosa* is possible, thus chlorinated swimming pools are not a risk but private jacuzzis or pools with inadequate disinfection should be avoided. Most *P. aeruginosa* infection is acquired outside hospital but *P. aeruginosa* is also found in hospital environments including washbasins and sinks.

Cross-infection with *P. aeruginosa* is rare but can occur, particularly with close and frequent contact between CF patients. A large 3-year study of 835 bacteriological samples from 72 unrelated CF patients and 22 siblings with CF showed that all unrelated patients were carrying different strains but siblings carried identical or closely related strains of *Pseudomonas*. Cross-infection has been shown between unrelated individuals attending the same holiday camp.

It is clear that there are some rare strains of *P. aeruginosa* that are more likely to cause cross-infectivity between patients (be transmissible) and there have been several reports of the same strain of *Pseudomonas* affecting CF patients in a CF centre, particularly those who had been staying in the same hospital ward. Respiratory secretions are the most likely source of transmission and efforts should be made to decrease the risk of transfer by segregating patients with known transmissible organisms and good general hygiene. It is important to remember that good handwashing and alcohol rubs remove *Pseudomonas*.

Transmission of organisms between patients has become an important issue in CF care and all sensible precautions should be taken. It is important however to keep a sense of perspective. Most organisms are acquired naturally in the community. Most isolations of *P. aeruginosa* are eradicated with early treatment. There is good evidence that regular attendance and follow-up at a specialist CF clinic is beneficial and is one of the major factors associated with increased lifespan in CF. Avoiding clinic attendance because of fear of infection is illogical and likely to be harmful in the long term.

Methicillin-resistant *Staphylococcus aureus* (MRSA)

Staphylococcus aureus is often the earliest and most common organism found in CF. Methicillin-resistant *S. aureus* (MRSA) is simply a form of the organism that has become resistant to a number of common antibiotics including methicillin. It is not surprising therefore that MRSA has appeared in CF at the same time as in non-CF patients, and that the prevalence in CF reflects the prevalence in the local community and hospital. MRSA was originally seen only in hospitals but is now widely disseminated and most infections are probably acquired in the community.

It appears that MRSA is more difficult to treat than a fully sensitive *S. aureus* and often a combination of antibiotics is required.

There have been a number of small trials of attempts to eradicate MRSA in CF. Eradication regimens consist of oral antibiotics combined with nasal creams and body and hair washes. High success rates can be achieved, but it has also been shown that about 50 per cent of CF patients will lose the organism over 6 months without any eradication attempts. CF patients with MRSA are kept separate from other patients in hospital.

Burkholderia cepacia (*B. cepacia*)

This organism was first identified as the cause of soft rot in onions and the first reports of isolations in CF individuals came in the 1970s. In the mid 1980s it became clear that some varieties of *B. cepacia* could cause a rapid severe and often fatal respiratory illness (cepacia syndrome) were resistant to many of the commonly used antibiotics and could spread from patient to patient by social contact. Intensive research over the past 20 years has clarified the situation.

Molecular analysis of isolates has revealed that there are at least 10 species of *B. cepacia*, some of which are almost entirely environmental and cause little lung disease on the rare occasions when they are found in CF. Accurate identification of a cepacia-like organism from a sputum sample is therefore very important and will usually need to be done in a specialized reference laboratory. Two species account for over 90 per cent of isolates from CF individuals in the UK: *B. cenocepacia* and *B. multivorans*. *B. cenocepacia* is often virulent and a particular substrain, ET10, is highly transmissible between patients. Current UK surveillance shows that the majority of new infection is by genetically distinct strains, i.e. individually acquired from the environment. Concern over possible transmission between patients means that all CF units segregate patients with *B. cepacia*-group organisms from other patients.

Other unusual organisms

There are a number of other unusual organisms that are occasionally identified from CF sputum, for example, *Stenotrophomonas maltophilia, Achromobacter* and *Ralstonia*. It is not clear how often these organisms add to the CF lung disease and they may simply be bystanders. They often clear without treatment.

Fungi

Aspergillus fumigatus is a common environmental organism. It is found in large quantities in mouldy hay and other decaying organic material and in small amounts everywhere from old buildings to pepper pots. It is frequently isolated from sputum or cough swabs and can occasionally cause direct airway damage (page 19). Some people with CF develop an allergic type of sensitivity to *Aspergillus* known as allergic bronchopulmonary aspergillosis. Other fungi cause problems in CF only rarely.

Atypical mycobacteria (non-tuberculous mycobacteria)

These are environmental mycobacteria which do not cause the disease tuberculosis – hence the term non-tuberculous mycobacteria. They can however be problematic in the cystic fibrosis lung and difficult to eradicate. There are many types but *Mycobacterium avium-intracellulare* (MAC) and *M. abscessus* are the two most commonly encountered in cystic fibrosis. They are most often found in older individuals.

9

Cystic fibrosis and the family

Konrad Jacobs & Louisa Demetriades

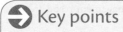 Key points

- Families with a child who has CF experience more stress

- Feeling well-informed about the condition tends to reduce stress

- Brothers and sisters can feel left out and jealous of the attention their parents give to the child with CF

- Adolescence is a difficult time for people with CF. The best strategy seems to be to acknowledge CF, do the treatment and get on with enjoying life

Living with cystic fibrosis and living with its treatment places great demands on every member of the family. This chapter describes some of the most common difficulties faced by families and offers ways of coping with and overcoming these difficulties.

Children with cystic fibrosis have a higher chance of developing emotional or behavioural difficulties (about twice as often) than children without CF. Many people feel that these numbers in fact reflect the extraordinary resilience of children with CF and their families: they face so many difficulties in life, and yet they only have a slightly higher chance of developing psychological difficulties!

Whether children (or their siblings and parents) experience any psychological difficulties is often not dependent upon the severity of the condition or any other disease-related factors, but much more on their and their family's *perceptions* of the situation, and the way they *cope* with it.

A number of factors make CF difficult for children. It is largely an 'invisible' condition and yet it places limitations upon children which other children do not have. It is also a condition with a strict treatment regimen, including physiotherapy, taking enzymes and using nebulizers, with no immediate 'reward' for this treatment. Children face an uncertain future, hospitalizations, and physical limitations. Adolescence can be particularly troublesome, as children may struggle with their identity formation and increased knowledge and awareness of their condition.

The next few paragraphs will briefly touch on some of the important issues to do with parents, adolescents with CF, siblings and self-management respectively.

Parents

Most people do not expect that their child will have a long-lasting medical condition. Parents' hopes and expectations for their children do not include CF. Some people bridge the gap between expectations and the reality very quickly, but others take a long time to come to terms with it. In the initial stages, parents may experience shock, denial, anger, guilt or depression. People usually do not experience these emotions in this particular order and often move from one emotion to another. Parents of children with CF may grieve the loss of the 'normal' child that they expected to have. In addition, parents may grieve the loss of the lifestyle that they expected for themselves and their family. Eventually, almost all parents reach an equilibrium and get on with the task of being a parent.

In some cases the diagnosis of CF has been missed for many years, and in those cases, parents may feel especially angry or depressed as their child has been suffering many symptoms for a long period of time without an apparent cause, and they find that ultimately one of their fears is in fact confirmed.

Knowledge of the condition helps parents at this stage. Feeling well-informed generally tends to reduce stress by providing a sense of control. On the other hand, it is easy to be overwhelmed by too much knowledge and each parent needs to find the level that suits them. Partners also differ in the amount of knowledge they want to hear.

Parental responsibilities in cystic fibrosis

- Finding out more about CF

- Dealing with your own emotions, which may include powerlessness, confusion, guilt, anger, frustration, fear, isolation, or depression

- Dealing with your children's' adjustment difficulties (your child with CF and its siblings)

- Dealing with uncertainty and fear about the future

- Coping with lifestyle changes (e.g. smoking)

- Financial implications

- Daily treatment regimen

- Dealing with your child's reluctance to keep undergoing treatment (non-compliance)

- Moving your child towards self-care

- What to tell your child about CF and when

- Time management

- Hospital appointments/hospitalization

- Building up positive relationships with the CF team

There are a number of roles and responsibilities parents of children with CF have over and above their normal parenting responsibilities. Some of these are summarized in the box below.

How does having a child with CF change family life and parenting? Families experience more stress than families of non-CF children. However, in general there is not much difference in child rearing or general family functioning. Parents of children with CF on the whole tend to be slightly more protective of their children and a little bit more controlling than parents of healthy children. This makes sense as parents of children with CF are naturally more concerned about their children's health and well-being than parents of non-CF children. Unfortunately, the flip side of 'protective' parenting is often that, paradoxically, children tend to become more anxious and more likely to show emotional or behavioural difficulties in the longer term. The challenge for parents (and indeed the wider family) is therefore to try to treat their CF children as normally as possible and have the same boundaries in place for their CF and their non-CF children.

Some parents may do the exact opposite: they act as much as possible as if nothing is happening. They do not want to talk about the condition, either because they feel it is not helpful or because it is hurtful. Sometimes people do not want to talk about difficulties because they think that other people will become upset if they do. They prefer to focus on the future and do not see the sense in focusing on something they cannot change. This reluctance to talk about a difficult subject is a very good strategy in some situations, but unfortunately not in others. It may protect people from feeling too overwhelmed by sadness or anger in the short term. On the other hand, in the longer term, it may lead to a culture within the family whereby difficult issues are not discussed. Also, not facing up to difficult issues is usually not an effective strategy in the long term: problems do not tend to go away by not thinking or talking about them and in fact they may fester and become worse. Open and sensitive discussion of difficult issues is usually most fruitful in the longer term.

The most commonly reported concerns by parents are the chronic burden of care, the life-shortening nature of the condition and disruptions in family relationships. With regard to marital relationships, the good news is that in general, there is no difference between partners with and without a child with a chronic illness in terms of marital satisfaction. Having said that, CF clearly increases stress related to the parenting role.

One of the most consistent findings is the fact that families that pull together, who are supportive, who communicate openly and positively tend to do better than families who do not do so.

To summarize: families experience more stress, but parental and family functioning is essentially no different from families of healthy children.

Adolescents

'When I was little I didn't really take note I had CF; it was just a thing and it was just part of my life just like anyone else has their own difficulties; it just wasn't a big thing; it was just part of your life and it never got in the way.'

Adolescence can be a particularly difficult period for children with CF. They gain more knowledge of their disease (sometimes more than they want to hear) and become more and more aware of the full implications of their condition, including their mortality. While their peers develop physically, their growth may be slow and the onset of puberty is often delayed. At the same time, they simply want to be 'normal', not any different from their peers, and are keen to become more independent from their parents to develop their individual identity.

Research that involved interviewing CF patients in their early teens provided a unique insight into the difficulties faced by these adolescents. Living with uncertainty was one of the key themes identified. They expressed uncertainty with regard to their symptoms (for example, feeling breathless raised uncertainty regarding what these symptoms meant), the trajectory of the illness course (what will happen as the disease progresses), the consequences of their symptoms (having to go to hospital or the life-limiting nature of the condition), and the possibility of and hope for a cure for CF.

The adolescents who were interviewed also described becoming gradually *more aware of the nature and implications of CF* from a scientific or medical perspective. However, their accounts clearly indicated that with such knowledge they also experienced a heightened awareness of their personal vulnerability, and this in turn often led to reluctance to learn more about the condition. They described a difficult balancing act between on the one hand a desire to find out more about their condition, and on the other hand a wish not to be overloaded by information and to control the emotional impact of the information. In clinic it is often clear that adolescents sometimes find out too much too quickly – via the Internet, for example – which can lead to anxiety, depression or treatment refusal.

Adolescents try to make sense of their *uniqueness*, the way they differ from their peers. It was often overwhelming for adolescents to deal with life, treatment and death issues to do with CF when their peers were going through 'normal' teenage development. Adolescents also found it difficult to deal with the increased visibility of their CF as a result of their physical under-development and delayed puberty. Many adolescents described feeling self-conscious about their differences from peers and identified this as 'the worst' aspect of their CF. Despite the unique challenges they were confronted with as a result of their CF, the adolescents talked about having good social lives and much-valued friendships.

A small number of the participants chose not to do any peer-related activities, such as going on school trips, in which others might become aware of their CF. However, most of the adolescents seemed to be aware that complete conceal-ment of their disease was both impossible and at times unhelpful. Telling oth-ers about their CF was often carefully planned. Thus, most of the adolescents told different details to people, with highly intimate personal information only to a selected few and less intimate information more widely revealed.

The final theme that emerged was about the importance of *acceptance* in ado-lescents with CF. Some adolescents described a big gap between how they would like to be and their actual situation. If they experienced this gap, they tended to be unhappy. Others stated that the best way to deal with CF was to acknowledge its presence, do the treatment and get on with enjoying life. This approach was related to less anxiety and depression.

The above themes show the kind of struggles adolescents face. It is there-fore not surprising that many adolescents go through rebellious or depressed phases or stages of refusing their treatment. A certain degree of distress is to be expected, and a normal part of the adjustment process. Most adolescents come out the other side. A minority will require a psychological intervention at this stage for continued distress.

Siblings

Siblings of children with CF are often a 'forgotten' group. They are in the unenviable position of having to watch their sibling suffer, being forced to join the condition's physical and emotional rollercoaster and not be able to affect its outcome. At the same time, professionals, and often parents as well, gener-ally do not pay as much attention to them as they do to the child with CF. Parents have reported treating their child with CF more leniently than their siblings, especially when that child was ill, and even children with CF reported that they felt that was the case. There is good and bad news for siblings of chil-dren with CF. On the negative side, they probably have a slightly raised chance of developing emotional or behavioural difficulties than children who are not in such a position, although not all studies show these results. However, simi-lar to children who actually have the condition, the resilience of this group of children is often remarkable.

More specifically, siblings may find some of the following issues difficult:

- ◆ Parents may treat the child with CF differently, for example sometimes the CF child may feel unwell, and parents may initially treat the child differently, e.g. excusing bad behaviour.

- Jealousy and feeling left out because of the amount of time parents spend with their brother or sister. Siblings subsequently often feel guilty or angry with themselves about feeling jealous. Williams (2001) put it as follows: '*I, as the well sibling, through no fault of anyone, often took a backseat to those who needed my parents' attention much more than I did ... as a child I felt left out.*'

- Embarrassment around peers.

- Feeling overly responsible for the emotional welfare or the self-management of their CF sibling.

- Concern regarding their parents' stress and grief.

- They may also struggle with some of the same issues as children with CF, e.g. how much to find out about CF, what to tell their friends, etc.

- Many siblings prefer to focus on the extent to which their brother or sister is 'normal' and just like other children and feel a great need to hold on to this image. They prefer not to talk about the illness.

On a more positive note, many children who have a sibling with a medical condition tend to be less self-centred and more appreciative of their own health. Having a sibling with a chronic life-threatening condition sometimes also improves their ability to empathize and cope with adversity.

Familial cohesion and support again work as buffers, protecting siblings from psychological distress. Siblings often want more information about what is happening to their brother or sister, guidance on their role and to feel that they too have a special place within the family.

Self-management

Most children with CF spend at least 1 hour per day on their treatment programme. The number of children who do all of their treatment (adherence) is notoriously low. Adherence to treatment has been estimated to be somewhere between 20 and 70 per cent, depending on the way it is measured and also depending on the treatment component. Chest physiotherapy and diet are the least adhered-to components of the treatment regimen whereas adherence to medication and vitamins is better. Adherence problems tend to increase with age, and peak in adolescence.

In the past, parents took full responsibility for all self-care aspects of cystic fibrosis, from very early on until well into the child's teenage years. This is no longer the accepted view. In an ideal world, children move smoothly through stages of ever-increasing control over their treatment and self-management towards full independence. On the other hand, too much independence too early on may lead to adherence problems in adolescence. There is a healthy middle ground with parents giving more and more control to their children, but at the same time remaining involved but increasingly in the background. It is of course not always easy to keep this balance. The establishment of a good treatment routine from early on is vital in this respect. Within a relatively strict routine, it is easier to pass more and more responsibility to the child.

Families who achieve shared responsibility, who listen to, encourage and support the child, and who experience low levels of serious conflict tend to have the least difficulties with non-compliance. However, most children and adolescents will experience hiccups along the way, and every person with CF will feel, at one time or another, that the challenge of self-care is a burden they want to escape. Personal characteristics and relationships influence how parents react to their children's non-compliance. Parents may become angry, controlling, or very insistent. They may try bribery, flattery, praise, talking, punishment or ignoring. One extreme reaction is what may be called the 'CF Police', where people try to control their child's CF completely, without reference to the child's wishes. In this situation, health takes a back seat to control. The first step in resolving the situation is to ask oneself the question: 'does what I am doing increase my child's compliance?' If the answer is 'no', a change of direction is needed. In many cases of child non-compliance, it is clear that parental behaviour, intended to help the child, often has the opposite effect and further entrenches the child. Any type of compulsion is likely to fail.

There are many possible reasons why children may stop complying. Sometimes, simple problem-solving can do the trick, for example if the child does not want to take enzymes in front of other children.

There is no immediate reward for doing any of the self-care activities. If somebody has a headache and takes an aspirin, the pain usually goes away fairly quickly. There is no such immediate 'reward' for children with CF who do their physiotherapy exercises. Many children either cannot take a longer-term perspective because they are too young, or they find it very difficult, as indeed do many adults. Children therefore often need external motivation for what they do in the form of praise and sometimes star or points charts.

Some children are keen to keep their parents' attention focused on them, whether it is positive or negative attention. They are often aware their parents are very keen for them to do their treatment, and therefore may decide that not cooperating is a good way to keep their parents involved with them.

In many cases, non-compliance is related to either too little or too much knowledge of the condition. Lack of knowledge is a surprisingly common reason for non-compliance. Younger children may not even know what CF is or why they are doing chest exercises every day. At the other end of the scale, children sometimes find out too much too quickly, particularly in their early teens. The knowledge may overwhelm them and they feel fatalistic about their condition: whatever they do, it is not going to make any difference.

Non-compliance can also be related to feeling 'different' and wanting to be 'normal'.

In general, if children feel relatively good about themselves, the people around them and their condition, there is no problem with compliance. As usual, communicating with children, sensitively exploring the reasons why the child finds treatment difficult is necessary to resolve the situation.

Conclusion

Cystic fibrosis is unexpected and unwanted. When a child is diagnosed with CF, the whole family is affected. Families who stick together and support each other tend to do better. Although children with CF, their siblings, and their families are under more stress most families function very well, and not any differently from families in which CF does not play a role. Most CF families lead happy lives. Difficulties and distress are to be expected in every family, and are normal as part of an adjustment process.

10

Cystic fibrosis and school

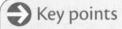 Key points

- Schools and teachers need to be told about the child with CF and how they can help

- Where possible the child with CF should not be treated differently from their schoolmates

- Children with CF should take part in all exercise activities

Entering school is a major new step for any child and parents are rightly concerned when there is additionally a medical problem such as cystic fibrosis. It is best to arrange to meet the teachers in advance and give then some information about CF and what it means for your child. Your local CF nurse may be able to come with you to help with this. Most teachers will not have encountered other children with CF, but most schools are extremely helpful once they have some understanding of the illness and how they can help.

Common issues at school

Enzymes

Most children have lunch at school, either a cooked school lunch or a packed lunch. Although it may be easier to provide a packed lunch so that you know what your child is eating (and how many enzymes they need) it is more important that your child is like the other children and is not an odd one out, e.g. the only one having a packed lunch. If they are having a cooked lunch then a best guess for enzymes is perfectly satisfactory – say, two enzyme capsules with a main course and one with a pudding.

It is important that there is a sensible arrangement for supervising your child taking their enzymes. For children starting at primary school, a dinner lady or teacher may be asked to check they are taking the enzymes. Some schools will wish to keep the enzymes and give them out at meal time. This may be satisfactory for a very young child, but in general it is a much better policy for the child to carry their enzymes either in their lunchbox or in an enzyme container in their pocket. Some schools are reluctant to permit this as they have rules about 'medications' and feel concerned that other children might swallow the capsules. It is often useful to regard and refer to enzymes as a food supplement rather than a drug and also useful to know that if another child swallowed the enzyme capsule there would be no ill effects – after all the child would only have a little more of enzymes they produce naturally. Remember that the child who has to go and ask for their enzymes is much less likely to take them and will be seen as different from their friends.

Healthy eating

There is considerable concern about children's diet and the increasing numbers of obese children. This has resulted in a campaign for healthy eating in schools and very often children are permitted only fruit and low-calorie drinks as snacks. For many children with CF this is perfectly satisfactory, but for those who have trouble gaining weight high-calorie snacks are to be encouraged. Once again the child will not want to be different from their friends, and compromises have to be reached such as a high-calorie fruit drink they bring to school rather than a squash drink.

Exercise

Most children with CF will be able, and should be encouraged, to take part in all activities with their contemporaries. Enough exercise to be out of breath is good for the lungs in CF. However, illness may result in loss of stamina and the teacher should be aware of this if, for example, the child has recently been off school with a lung infection.

Physiotherapy at school

It is rare for physiotherapy to be needed during the school day. However, there are some families where for social reasons physiotherapy is rarely given at home and in these special cases a school helper may be taught how to perform physiotherapy.

Mixing with other individuals who have cystic fibrosis

Occasionally there is more than one child with cystic fibrosis in a school and rarely there may be a teacher with it. It is sensible to avoid close contact but not to restrict casual contact, i.e., not to be in same classroom all day every day but to take part in normal mixing in playgrounds.

Academic ability

Cystic fibrosis does not affect brain power, and children with CF are as academically able as others in their class. They may, however, have to miss time from school with infections or other illnesses and at such times may need some extra help to catch up. If someone is unlucky enough to have had significant illness during preparations for formal examinations then examination boards should be informed and will take this into consideration.

 Patient's perspective

Justine is 17 and is someone who was unlucky enough to run into major problems early in life. She gave this talk at a conference and has given us permission to print it in full.

My journey with CF

Hello, I've been asked to talk about living with a life-limiting illness and what I feel has and hasn't helped me so far.

I was born with cystic fibrosis, which has a life expectancy of around 30. The main problem in CF is the overproduction of thick, sticky mucus which clogs the lungs and digestive system. My stomach is easy to manage, but my lungs became very badly damaged due to constant chest infections, which became harder to treat.

I thought it would be helpful to firstly summarize the main stages of my illness and the treatment I have undergone.

My first operation was at birth, when I suffered a bowel blockage, meconium ileus, which had to be removed. Once home, the start of intense treatment began, with more as I got older.

From the start, chest physiotherapy to help remove any mucus from my lungs and from the age of 3, nebulized antibiotics to reduce infection.

At the age of 6, my chest began to deteriorate, so I started having regular courses of around-the-clock intravenous antibiotics through long lines in my arms. As this went on, vein access became harder so I had my first portacath inserted when I was 8 and had another two subsequently due to blockages and leaks.

At the age of 9, I developed pneumonia; my right lung partially collapsed and would not re-inflate because of a mass of infection in my right lower lobe. After weeks of intense treatment the lobe was removed by a lobectomy in May 2000. This was done at the John Radcliffe Hospital, which is currently my CF centre.

My chest was never the same after that and was gradually getting worse. The amount of treatment too was becoming more frequent and I was beginning to feel more breathless whenever I did anything. Everyday tasks I couldn't manage like climbing stairs or even washing my hair. I had a CT scan done which revealed severe lung damage. At this point doctors told my parents that a lung transplant may be an option in the next couple of years.

Two years later when I was 12, although transplantation was never mentioned to me by anyone, I knew about it and discreetly did research on the Internet to see if it was something that I wanted to undergo and decided that it was. My local doctors then referred me to Great Ormond Street Hospital for transplant assessment in November 2002. I was accepted, but asked to wait until after Christmas. I was put on the active list in January 2003.

In February that year, I started another course of IV antibiotics but due to an allergic reaction to the drugs I suffered acute renal failure. I was rushed to Great Ormond Street to start peritoneal dialysis which lasted for 1 month. I was very sick, resulting in me being suspended from the transplant list.

It took my body a long time to recover from what was such a huge shock. Once I had, tests revealed that probably due to the levels of antibiotics in my system from the renal failure this killed the majority of infection which resulted in a better lung function. I actually seemed to be keeping slightly better and didn't need IV's for the next 10 months. It was therefore decided that I should not be placed back on the transplant list at that point. But the following year, 2004 things started to deteriorate as none of this has ever fixed my lung damage and my lung function dropped again.

On the 16th of November, 2 days after my 14th birthday, I was placed back on the list.

Life remained the same as there were no guarantees and we were just focusing on keeping me as well as possible for an operation that could possibly happen at any time.

In April 2005, we had just arrived back from our holiday home in Devon when in the early hours of the following morning I was called for my transplant.

That day I became Great Ormond Street's 100th double lung transplant patient. Because of this I have been asked to speak for them at several press events.

After a long recovery period and the addition of a few new problems, namely a deep vein thrombosis, diabetes and a 9-month period of physical sickness due to a steroid imbalance connected to my adrenal suppression, my life in terms of treatment and breathing has changed considerably and finally for the better.

To illustrate what has and hasn't helped me, I thought it would be easier to put my life into three main areas: hospital, school and home.

First to hospital and what has helped.

Most of my treatment was home-based. This was only possible due to the fantastic support and friendship of the paediatric Hospital-at-Home team, who work at Wycombe General Hospital. They came out on numerous visits, sometimes out of hours to teach mum how to administer IV drugs and work equipment. They were not always the easiest of visits, especially when I wasn't the most compliant patient, but we always ended up having a laugh however difficult things had been! If it had not been for them, I would have spent a lot more of my life in hospital.

I feel very lucky to have had a very supportive consultant both at Wycombe and Oxford who I know have always done their best for me. They never questioned when we felt I needed IVs.

My mum and I have a very good friend on the Iain Rennie Hospice-At-Home team who has always been there to help us when we have needed it and still keeps in touch with us regularly now – nothing is ever too much trouble for her.

Now for what hasn't helped!

The different doctors who come in and ask for medical history and what drugs I am on when my notes are there in front of them. I didn't always feel well enough to keep going through everything and they didn't always have the best bedside manner.

Doctors who clearly can't take blood and waste a vein when they are already damaged.

Doctors who don't listen or underestimate a problem just because I have had a transplant. Problems do still occur and a patient knows their body best!

Play specialists who try to help when really they are not. They don't distract a teenager who knows exactly what is going on. Even when I was younger, bubbles didn't help!

Now to school. Both my infant and junior schools were very understanding and flexible, even though the major problems didn't arise until I was in senior school.

I am very lucky to have my senior school very close to home, which accommodates children with special needs and is all on one level, which meant I had no stairs to climb.

There is a resident full-time qualified matron who has been a huge support to me pre- and post-transplant. I was only able to attend school part time and even then often had to rest either in her ward or go home. I was given a pass which enabled me to be late to lessons, leave a lesson early and access any part of the school if it gave me a shortcut due to my breathing difficulties. She has made my schooling much easier to deal with and she would always sort out any problems with teachers. She has become a very close friend and I believe every school should have a qualified matron.

Now for what hasn't helped!

The lack of continuity between teachers. This meant I could walk into a lesson to have a teacher who knew nothing about my circumstances. They also never helped me to catch up with any work that I had missed due to long absences.

I found it hard to get into a group of friends as they too didn't understand my situation. I was often accused of being miserable as I could not take part in anything, and this made me really angry as nobody knew what I was going through and that it was my illness that was holding me back.

And finally, what has helped in home life.

Equipment being built in at home. I had an oxygen concentrator which I had to go on every night, a chair lift, so I didn't have to climb the stairs. I also had a wheelchair to go out in. I hardly ever went out because I didn't want to be seen in it, but it was there if I needed it and there were times where I didn't have a choice, such as hospital trips where it was useful.

My pets. I used to say that I couldn't go out into the world therefore I had to bring the world to me, which was through getting more animals. My first dog Monty was with me throughout the really low points and I found him a real comfort, especially at the times when my illness got me down. He was with me since birth to my transplant and died 6 months after that, so he was my lifelong friend. Animals don't judge you and love you for who you are, however you are.

Lastly, my close family, my mum, dad and older sister. In their own individual way, they have all been a huge support for me and I know that without them I would not have come through the tragic times that I have. I know that I don't always show my appreciation as I would be the first to admit I am not and have not been the easiest person to live with, but that has never stopped them all caring for me and for that I will always be grateful to them. Something that causes tension in home life is the fact that my sister and I have the same condition. It is very rare that we are both well at the same time. Before my transplant, it was me who held everyone back. Now Jacqueline's health is more unstable which causes friction between us. Everyone always assumes that we have a close bond because we have the same illness, but that isn't the case. I admit that it is me who is more intolerant especially since my transplant. As far as the wider family are concerned, at the really toughest of times, you realize who your family are. There is a huge truth in the saying 'When the going gets tough, the tough get going'.

My transplant has made a huge difference to my quality of life. I have been able to be much more independent. It has enabled me to have a full time education, and take my GCSEs last June without long disruptions. I am now able to go out with friends, take part in activities that I enjoy and had a Saturday job at a hairdressing salon back in summer. Most noticeably, the amount of treatment is now hugely reduced. No IVs, physiotherapy or nebulizers. As this speech is partly about what has helped, this transplant certainly has, therefore I feel a special mention is for my donor family, who were able to make the decision to donate organs. Without them, I would probably not be standing here today talking to you all. A thank you will never be enough to match what they have done for me, as they have given me the gift of a better quality of life, something which I will always treasure.

I also want to use this occasion to acknowledge the highly skilled and dedicated teams involved in my care. They have done a fantastic job.

I don't ever think about what the future holds for me. During my life with CF I have heard of and seen people pass away with this same illness and who did not manage to get their transplant in time. Therefore, I count myself extremely lucky to have survived all the horrific challenges life has thrown at me and what I have been given. I will enjoy life as fully as I can and achieve what I want to do. I am a great believer in positive thinking and a sense of humour will get you through anything. The body will never give up until the mind does.

I hope that I have raised awareness at this conference about how things make a difference, both good and bad, to young people and their families who are living with a life-limiting condition, and hope that certain areas could be addressed in the future, just to make life that little bit easier.

Thank you for listening.

11

Growing up with cystic fibrosis

> ## ➔ Key points
>
> ◆ Transition to adult care should occur gradually at a pace governed by the young person with CF
>
> ◆ Cystic fibrosis has no effect on sexual function but it does affect fertility
>
> ◆ The results of lung transplantation are improving: 75 per cent of adults survive more than 2 years and 50 per cent more than 5 years after transplantation

The outlook for people with cystic fibrosis has been transformed over the past 20 years. Cystic fibrosis is still a life-shortening disease but in 2006 there are now more adults with cystic fibrosis in the UK than there are children.

As children grow up and enter their teens they wish to have more independence from their parents. It is important to try to ensure that cystic fibrosis treatment does not become a battleground between the teenager and their parents. If possible it is best from very early on to allow the young person to have individual responsibility for their treatment which increases with time. A good example would be learning some of the components of the active cycle of breathing physiotherapy technique from the age for 7 or 8 years, and gradually increasing the responsibility for physiotherapy so that the child is fully independent from his or her parents by the age of 12 or 13. Parental help is then reserved for times of exacerbations.

Transition to adult care

The transition from paediatric to adult care can be a difficult time for the young person and their parents. The age at which this happens most comfortably will vary from person to person. In general it should be sometime between the age of 16 and 19 years (or between 18 and 21 in the US) depending on the physical and emotional maturity of the young person. It is important that in advance of a move to an adult clinic there are opportunities to meet members of the adult team, which may include joint transition clinics or hospital visits and in particular getting to know the adult cystic fibrosis nurse, who will be a very important contact person. A natural time for transition is very often around the age of 17–18 years when other transitions to college or university or the workplace also occur. In general transition is much more difficult for parents than for the young person with cystic fibrosis.

Cystic fibrosis and work

Most adults with cystic fibrosis are either in full-time education or work. It is sensible to plan for an occupation that is not physically demanding. It is best to tell an employer about the illness and under Disability Discrimination legislation an employer is obliged to make 'reasonable adjustments' for a person with a disability, which includes CF. This might include being flexible about working hours and allowing time off for medical appointments.

Puberty, sex, fertility and pregnancy

Puberty may occur later in individuals with cystic fibrosis (as it does in any chronic disease) thus girls may not start their periods till around 14 years and boys not reach final height till 16 or 17 years.

Cystic fibrosis has no effect on sexual function in men or women but does affect fertility.

Most men with cystic fibrosis are infertile because the tube which carries sperm from the testes to the penis (the vas deferens) became blocked many years before puberty and has disappeared (absence of vas deferens). Some men with very mild CF symptoms are only diagnosed when seen at an infertility clinic. Women have normal ovaries and womb and can produce healthy eggs but if they are underweight they may have irregular menstrual cycles.

If men with cystic fibrosis wish to have children there is a technique available where, under local anaesthetic, sperm are taken directly from the epididymus or testes and injected into eggs taken from the female partner. This technique is called intercytoplasmic sperm injection (ICSI). Fertilized eggs are then returned to the woman's uterus so that they can develop normally. About one in four such attempts are successful.

Women are fertile but should consider the possible effects on their health before embarking on pregnancy. Women with good lung function and good health usually have a successful pregnancy. Lung function decreases by about 13 per cent during pregnancy but most of that can be regained afterwards. It is important to have good health care during pregnancy.

Before embarking on pregnancy anyone with CF will wish to consider the long-term impact of their condition on their children's life.

Complications

The long-term complications such as osteoporosis and diabetes discussed in Chapter 4 become more frequent during adult life and add to an already complicated treatment regimen.

Respiratory failure

As lung disease in CF progresses it becomes more difficult to transfer gases through the lung into and out of the bloodstream. The levels of oxygen in the blood fall and the levels of carbon dioxide in the blood increase. Breathing becomes more difficult during activity and eventually even at rest. The low levels of oxygen and higher levels of carbon dioxide in the blood eventually have an effect on the heart and blood vessels. There is gradual development of increased blood pressure in the blood vessels of the lungs. This is known as pulmonary hypertension. In turn pulmonary hypertension leads to strain on the heart as it is harder for the heart to deliver blood to the lungs.

The oxygen level in the blood is measured using an oxygen saturation machine with a finger or ear probe. Individuals who are developing respiratory problems may at first need some oxygen at night time and on exercise. As the disease progresses they may also need oxygen for daily activities. If the level of carbon dioxide in the bloodstream at night time is high the individual may have morning headaches, morning nausea and take several hours before they feel back to their normal self. Sometimes using a breathing machine at night time will decrease the effort of breathing at night, improve sleep and make the individual feel better in the morning. This is known as non-invasive ventilation, as the individual triggers the breathing machine by wearing a nasal mask.

Lung transplantation

When it is clear that an individual has severe lung disease which is irreversible and it is affecting their life – long periods off school or work, unable to walk without oxygen, etc. – it is time to discuss lung transplantation. Not everyone with CF wishes to go forward for transplantation but most will want to investigate and understand the process before making a decision.

There are only a limited number of centres which perform lung transplantation. Generally an individual will be referred by their CF doctor to one of the centres for evaluation. The evaluation is rather like an annual review with an emphasis on how much the person can do, their lung function and assessment of things that may make transplantation more difficult, for example infection with *Burkholderia cenocepacia* or previous lung surgery. The process and surgery is explained in detail so the individual can think it through and discuss with family and friends before making a decision on whether to proceed.

Types of transplant
Heart–lung transplant

The earliest transplants were of both heart and lungs. The heart and lungs were removed in a block from the patient with CF and the heart then made available for transplant to another individual with heart disease. Thus the procedure was known as a domino transplant. The reason for transplanting both heart and lungs was that it was a technically easier procedure for the surgeon.

Double lung transplant

In this procedure the cystic fibrosis lungs are removed one by one and replaced by donor lungs.

Single lung transplant

In some individuals it is only possible to transplant one lung. This may be because one lung had been removed previously or there was a specific abnormality of the chest. Both cystic fibrosis lungs are removed and a single healthy donor lung transplanted.

Live donor two-lobe transplants

This is a technique where a part (lobe) of a lung from two live donors is transplanted. One donor gives a lobe from the right lung and another a lobe from the left lung. This involves risk for both donors and so far has not been very successful. It remains experimental.

 FAQ

How successful is transplantation?

Results are improving as new anti-rejection drugs become available. In adults 5 per cent will die in the immediate post-operative time;

75 per cent survive more than 2 years and 50 per cent are still alive 5 years after transplantation.

What happens after transplantation?

Once the patient is discharged from hospital they are kept under very close follow-up. They have to take anti-rejection drugs for the rest of their life. Patients are asked to monitor their lung function on a daily basis and to alert the transplantation centre if there is any variation. The greatest hazard is for rejection of the new lungs. A type of chronic rejection known as bronchiolitis obliterans is the most common long-term problem.

Death

Cystic fibrosis is a life-shortening disease. Despite the best of treatments the disease progresses and near the end of life some individuals will be waiting for a lung transplant and others will have decided it is not for them. When considering this issue it is best to be able to talk to someone about the process of death. There is usually a member of the CF team who has become close and feels comfortable to talk to. Many people wish to die at home and the team will give all their support to allow this to happen. For others the hospital CF unit or a familiar hospice is the right place for them and where they feel supported. Symptoms of breathlessness, discomfort or anxiety are relieved by morphine-based drugs so the patient can be awake enough to communicate with their loved ones and in due course gradually die in sleep. Many people will have made clear the arrangements they wish for funerals and have created memory boxes to share and leave with their families.

 Patient's perspective

Jemma's statement when in hospital with a chest infection:

I'm 16 and have cystic fibrosis. Living with CF can be tiring and twice-a-day physiotherapy doesn't help. But if doing physio and taking all sorts of tablets means your chest is clear and you have loads of energy, you would do it wouldn't you? If you were sensible, yes you would! But I wasn't. As soon as I hit the teenage years, I acted like any normal teenage girl.

12

Future therapies

 Key points

- There is very active research on new therapies for CF

- Approaches include trying to correct the basic defect by adjusting the CFTR protein; carrying normal CFTR into cells (gene therapy); and restoring the transfer of salts across the cell membrane (ion transport)

- Improving current treatments and making them work better is also likely to have real benefits in the near future

It is very likely that there will be new therapies for cystic fibrosis in the future. The medical research funding bodies across the world including the CF charities are funding academic research essential for the understanding of the disease process and are working in partnership with pharmaceutical companies to develop new drugs.

The CF trust in the UK has concentrated research funding on developing gene therapy. The Cystic Fibrosis Foundation in the USA and other national research funding bodies support a variety of approaches to tackle the disease at different points (Figure 12.1).

There are stringent regulations for bringing a new drug to market, controlled in the USA by the Food and Drug Administration (FDA) and in Europe by the European Medicines Agency (EMEA). Before pharmaceutical companies start trials on humans extensive pre-clinical studies are carried out in the laboratory and in animal models. Trials on humans are conducted in three phases.

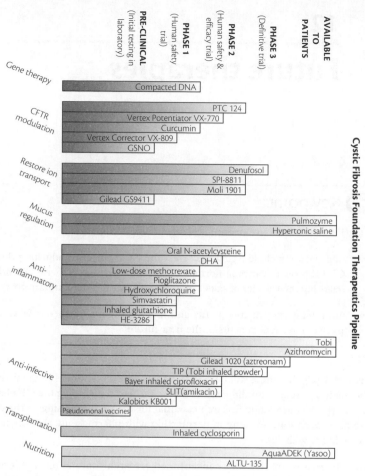

Figure 12.1 Cystic Fibrosis Foundation timeline for new therapies (DHA, docosahexaenoic acid; GSNO, 5-nitroso-glutathione). Reproduced with permission of the CFF.

Clinical studies

Phase 1 studies

This is the earliest stage after laboratory tests have shown that the new treatment might be useful. Phase 1 studies are conducted in small numbers of volunteers (20–80) and are designed to find out:

- whether the drug is safe to use

- the safe dose range

- the side-effects

- how the body copes with the drug.

Phase 2 studies

If the drug is considered safe in phase 1 trials it proceeds to a phase 2 study. Here it is tested in larger numbers of people (100–300) to examine how effective it is as well as to confirm its safety. Many drugs fail at this stage because toxic side-effects are discovered or the drug does not seem to work as well as expected.

Phase 3 studies

Phase 3 studies involve large numbers of patients and are designed to compare the new drug with current therapies. This often involves a double-blind randomized controlled trial. Double-blind means that neither the patient nor the doctor knows whether the patient is taking the real drug or a dummy one until the trial is finished. These trials are very expensive and difficult to run, especially in chronic conditions like CF.

Once the drug has been shown to be effective in phase 3 studies then the manufacturer submits all the information to the regulatory authorities for approval to sell the drug. Drug companies are granted tax benefits and other government subsidies to help develop drugs (orphan drugs) for rare diseases such as CF (orphan diseases) in both USA and Europe. This is important as otherwise it would be too expensive for the drug company to bring their products to market.

Main areas of research

Restoring ion transport

The purpose is to correct the defect on the surface of the cells lining the airways (epithelial cells) so that the depth and salt concentration of the liquid layer on the surface of the cells returns to normal. The cilia should then be able to clear mucus more efficiently from the lungs. The drugs being investigated act on chloride and/or sodium channels across the cell wall. Some of the drugs have been shown to be very effective in the very short term, but the challenge is to find a drug or combination of drugs which will act to restore the depth of airway surface liquid for long periods.

Anti-inflammatory drugs

Inflammation in the lung increases as the disease progresses. It is known that drugs with anti-inflammatory properties are helpful in CF, for example oral steroids or ibruprofen, but their use is limited by side effects. A number of other drugs, some of which are already available for use in other diseases, are being trialled for usefulness and safety in CF.

Anti-infective agents

New types of antibiotics, that work in different ways from those currently available, are being developed. Also, antibiotics already used in CF are being altered to allow them to be used in a different way e.g. aztreonam currently used intravenously is being developed for use through a nebulizer. Work on a *Pseudomonas* vaccine continues. There is also work looking at ways to stimulate the body's natural protection against *Pseudomonas*.

Adjusting the CFTR protein (CFTR modulation)

As explained in Chapter 13, the different gene defects effect the production, transport and processing of CFTR protein in different ways. A number of drugs are being developed to try to bypass the defect, or to permit more of the CFTR protein to reach the cell surface.

Mucus clearance

Drugs such as hypertonic saline have been shown to aid mucus clearance in selected patients with CF. Further studies in which groups of patients benefit from hypertonic saline are under way. Another drug, Lomucin (talniflumate), which decreases mucus production has also been studied.

Making current treatment easier to use

Another area of research is finding simpler and quicker ways of delivering current therapies.

There is continuing work on nebulizer technology:

♦ to increase the proportion of drug reaching the lung

♦ to predict which part of the lung is reached by the drug

♦ to adjust the nebulizer characteristics to reach different parts, i.e. titrate the nebulizer to the patient.

There is work on converting drugs currently delivered by nebulizer to a form in which they can be delivered by inhaler, e.g. colomycin and tobramycin.

Gene therapy

The idea is that if a normal *CFTR* gene can be inserted into the airway cell then the basic defect could be corrected. There have been a number of small trials using parts of viruses or other agents to carry the gene into cells in the nose or lungs and these have demonstrated that gene transfer is possible in principle and that partial correction of the defect can be achieved. However, when viruses were used as the carriers there was evidence that they produced inflammation so were not suitable for long-term use. Other non-viral agents such as lipids are now being used in addition to modified viruses.

There are many hurdles to overcome including getting sufficient amounts of the replacement gene to the correct place; making sure it can work for some weeks before further treatment is needed; and making sure there is no evidence of toxicity or side effects. Although on paper the gene therapy approach to correcting CF appears the easiest it may be the most difficult to make effective.

The CFF in the US is supporting the development of a non-viral *CFTR* replacement product delivered to the lung in compacted DNA particles. This is in a phase 1 study.

The CF Trust in the UK funds the Gene Therapy Consortium, a group of scientists based in Edinburgh, London and Oxford who together have developed non-viral gene transfer systems. They have also been optimizing nebulizer delivery systems for gene products and trying to establish the best ways to assess the effectiveness of gene therapy. They are currently (in 2008) recruiting 200 patients to pursue a phase 2 trial.

13

Genetics of cystic fibrosis

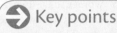 **Key points**

- Cystic fibrosis is an autosomal recessive disorder

- The gene responsible for CF is called the cystic fibrosis transmembrane conductance regulator (*CFTR*) and is located on the long arm of chromosome 7

- More than 1500 errors (mutations) causing CF have been discovered in the *CFTR* gene. The most common is called *Delta F508*

Every part of the human body is made up of millions of cells. These cells are too small to be seen by the naked eye, but they can be looked at through a microscope in which they are magnified maybe 50 to 100 times. Each cell works as an independent machine that also talks to its neighbours to make the body function as an integrated whole. All the cells of an individual have the same genetic information. It is this information that is responsible for the inherited characteristics of an individual.

Body cells are continually dividing during life; in this way the body can grow and repair itself. When a cell divides, it produces two daughter cells, each of which contains the same genetic information as the parent cell. To achieve this, the parental cell genetic information is duplicated before cell division so that there are two sets of this information, one for each daughter cell.

The genetic material is contained within structures called chromosomes (see Figure 13.1) which have a short (p) arm and a long (q) arm separated by a central constriction, the centromere.

Different species have different numbers of chromosomes. Humans normally have 46 chromosomes in all the cells of their body apart from the sex cells (the eggs or the sperm). Each of these body cells is diploid, i.e. it carries two complete sets of genetic information. Thus the 46 chromosomes consist of two sets of 23.

One chromosome set comes from the mother via the ovum (egg) and the other comes from the father via the particular sperm that fertilized the ovum. Both ovum and sperm are haploid, that is they carry only a single set of 23 chromosomes. When egg and sperm fuse in fertilization, the chromosome complement of the ensuing embryo is restored to 46 (23 pairs).

In 22 of these 23 pairs of chromosomes, members of the pair are the same in men and women. These pairs are known as the autosomes. The twenty-third pair comprises the sex chromosomes, X and Y. Women have two X chromosomes, men have one X chromosome and one Y. Unlike the autosome pairs, the X and Y chromosomes are functionally dissimilar. The Y chromosome is very small in comparison with the X and apparently carries very little genetic information, apart from that required to direct male sexual development.

As has already been mentioned, the ovum and the sperm only carry a single set of chromosomes. Eggs and sperm are made by a process called meiosis: a diploid cell with 46 chromosomes divides into haploid cells containing 23 chromosomes each. If meiosis simply involved one chromosome from each pair going into each haploid cell, then the maternal and paternal chromosomes would remain unchanged from generation to generation and there would be little genetic diversity. What actually happens is that during meiosis the two sets of genetic information in the cell are shuffled like two packs of cards. This process is known as recombination.

Before the cell divides in meiosis, the chromosomes join in homologous pairs. This means that chromosome 1 inherited from the mother joins up with the corresponding paternal chromosome, and likewise chromosome 2, 3, 4, etc. pair up. Random and reciprocal exchanges of genetic material then occur within each homologous pair, involving sections of genetic material from one chromosome breaking off and replacing the equivalent section on the other chromosome (see Figure 13.1).

The two main chemical components of chromosomes are deoxyribonucleic acid (DNA) and proteins. It is the DNA that within its structure contains all the information needed to construct a human being from a single fertilized egg. Each DNA molecule can replicate itself, making an identical copy of its genetic information. However, for this genetic information to be useful to the cell, it must be translated into a form that can be used by the cell machinery

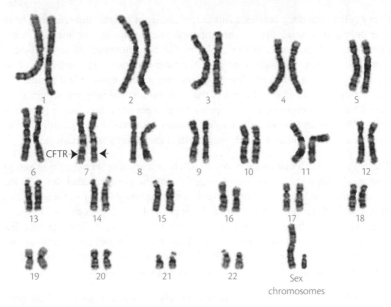

Figure 13.1 The chromosomes of a normal human male. The banding pattern, produced using a special stain, is characteristic of each pair of chromosomes. The CF gene is located halfway down the long (q) arm of chromosome 7. Courtesy of Katrin M Carlson, Ph.D., Director, Cytogenetics, Children's Memorial Hospital, Chicago, USA.

outside the nucleus. To achieve this the DNA has to be copied, or transcribed, into another molecule called ribonucleic acid (RNA), which is further processed to generate messenger RNA. In turn, this messenger RNA is used as a blueprint for the translation of the genetic message into biologically useful molecules, i.e. proteins.

Proteins are made up of a long chain of building blocks, called amino acids. The chemical sequence in the RNA copy of the DNA directs the insertion of a particular amino acid in a specific place in each protein. There are 20 different types of amino acid with different biochemical properties which perform the functions of a protein and many thousands of different proteins are made in the one cell. Proteins can really be regarded as the primary product of genetic information and all the different proteins made in an individual are responsible for his or her uniqueness. They have a wide range of functions in the body: structural proteins are major components of muscle, skin, hair, and many other tissues, while enzymes are essential parts of the body's metabolism.

Every cell in the body carries a full complement of genetic information, however only a very small part of this information is used in any one cell at any one time. In fact, much of the DNA in the chromosomes is never used in coding for proteins, though some of it has other functions. The important coding regions of the DNA are found within functional units called genes. It is the coding regions within the genes that are transcribed into messenger RNA which then goes on to be the blueprint for protein manufacture, as described above. Within and between genes or groups of genes are large non-coding regions of DNA, some of which may control the activity of specific genes.

The cells of a particular tissue or organ will have a specific set of genes in action. Hence, although the enzyme-secreting cells of the pancreas and the cells lining the airway will have certain active genes in common – that is, those making products that are essential for the maintenance of any living cell – other active genes will be coding for products involved in tissue-specific functions. For example, the pancreas secretory cells will have active genes producing specific digestive enzymes to break down food, while genes coding for mucus will be switched on in many of the cells lining the respiratory tract.

It should be remembered here that each cell contains a pair of each gene, one from each parent. Genes coding for the same product can vary slightly in their precise DNA sequence from one person to the next. Where an individual has inherited identical forms (alleles) of a particular gene from both parents he is said to be homozygous for that gene, but if he has inherited non-identical alleles for any specific gene he is defined as heterozygous for that gene. The words heterozygote and carrier of a particular gene are interchangeable.

Genetic diseases, also called inherited diseases, are caused by abnormal genes that do not fulfil their proper function. An abnormal gene can be classed as dominant or recessive. If an abnormal gene is dominant, its abnormality is manifest even if the other gene of the pair is normal. However, when an abnormal gene is recessive, the abnormality is masked if the other gene of the pair is normal. Cystic fibrosis is a recessive genetic disease, so in order to have the illness a child has probably inherited defective genes from both its parents. New errors in the genetic information only arise rarely, so usually both parents of a CF baby are heterozygous for CF – that is, they have one normal and one abnormal gene – and are known as a carriers of the abnormal gene. Carriers do not have the symptoms of the disease, but may pass it on to their offspring.

The combination of all the different genes that an individual has are known as his or her genotype. Simple inheritance patterns of dominant and recessive genes are illustrated in Figure 13.2, and the classical inheritance pattern of the CF gene from two carrier parents is shown in Figure 13.3.

Both dominant and recessive diseases can be subdivided into autosomal and sex-linked conditions, which are coded for by genes located on the autosomes or on the sex chromosomes, respectively. The known inheritance pattern of the CF gene, derived from the study of many affected families, shows that equal numbers of male and female CF children are born to healthy parents. From this pattern it is clear that the CF gene must be autosomal and not sex-linked. Recessive diseases coded for by a gene on the X chromosome, such as haemophilia, are much more common in males than in females. This is because a male has only one X chromosome, so there is no possibility of

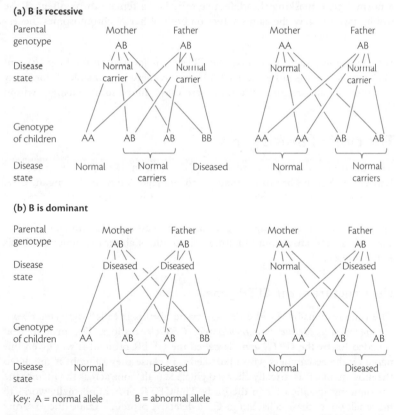

Key: A = normal allele   B = abnormal allele

Figure 13.2 Diagram to illustrate dominant and recessive inheritance if (a) abnormal allelle B is recessive, and (b) if abnormal allele B is dominant.

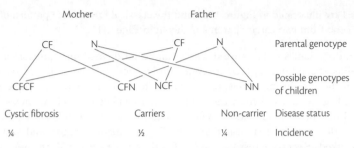

Figure 13.3 Inheritance of the CF gene from two carrier parents. Key: CF, CF gene; N, normal gene.

a normal gene masking the defective one. For a female to be affected she would have to carry the same defect on both of her X chromosomes, necessarily a rare event.

We have known since 1985 that the CF gene is located on the long (q) arm of chromosome 7 (see Figure 13.1). However, there is no visible abnormality in chromosome structure; the faults are much more subtle changes within the DNA.

The cystic fibrosis gene

The isolation of the cystic fibrosis (CF) gene in 1989 by the groups of Lap-Chee Tsui in Toronto, Canada, and Francis Collins in Michigan, USA was a tremendous achievement at the time and built on the work of several research teams over the preceding 10 or more years. Isolation of the gene opened a new and exciting chapter in CF research. It was now possible to start asking and answering fundamental questions about the molecular basis of the disease.

The structure of the *CFTR* gene

The gene responsible for the disease cystic fibrosis is called the *cystic fibrosis transmembrane conductance regulator* – *CFTR* for short. The protein that is coded for by the *CFTR* gene is called the CFTR protein. It was given this name by the researchers who identified it because they thought it regulated the movement of electrically charged chloride (salt) ions across the membrane surrounding specific cells in the body. The CFTR protein normally works to move salt out of these cells, but in CF a defective protein is made due to errors in the *CFTR* gene and so normal chloride movement cannot take place.

The *CFTR* gene is large, spanning about 190 000 units of genetic information on the long arm of chromosome 7. In fact only a small part of this genetic information, 6200 units, actually codes for the message that directs the making of the CFTR protein. The coding region of the *CFTR* gene is made up of 27 individual units that are copied from the DNA of the gene and joined to each other in a chain (messenger RNA). The coding region directs the assembly of a protein containing 1480 amino acids, called the CFTR protein.

What does the CFTR protein do?

The CFTR protein probably looks something like the illustration in Figure 13.4. It appears to be anchored within the membrane surrounding the cells in which it is found and to form a pore in that membrane through which electrically charged chloride ions can pass out of the cell. The pore in the cell membrane is normally closed but when chloride needs to move out of the cell the CFTR protein changes shape to allow the pore to open.

Though it is now certain that the movement of chloride through the pore in the cell membrane is one function of the CFTR protein, we now know that the protein has additional functions. For example, it interacts with other proteins that move different types of salt in and out of cells and influences their activity. Thus, in the layer of cells lining the airway, absence of normal CFTR protein causes the protein that moves sodium salts into the cells to be hyperactive. This secondary effect of errors in CFTR is fundamental to CF airway disease.

Where is the CFTR protein found?

As with many other important proteins that carry out highly specialized functions, the CFTR protein is not found in all cell types and organs in the body. Expression of the *CFTR* gene in readily detectable amounts appears to be largely restricted to the layer of cells (called epithelial cells) that line certain organs. The majority of these cell layers are within the ducts of the organs, for example the pancreatic ducts, the sweat gland ducts, and the male genital ducts. CFTR protein is also found in parts of the layer of cells that lines the small and large intestine. This pattern of expression of the CFTR protein is perhaps to be expected, since these are all tissues that are affected by the CF disease process. Surprisingly, given the central role of the lung in CF, there is relatively little expression of the CFTR protein in the layer of cells that lines the airways and the lungs, with only a few cell types having the protein. Since we know that the CF disease process has already started before birth, while the baby is still in the uterus, it was of interest to see where the CFTR protein is found in the developing fetus. The main surprise was that in the middle of pregnancy there is apparently plenty of CFTR protein within the layer of cells that lines the airways and lungs, but this gradually declines as gestation proceeds. This may be important in CF lung disease, but we do not yet understand how. There remain many gaps, such as this, in our understanding of how exactly the CF disease process happens.

Errors (mutations) in the *CFTR* gene

Over the past 18 years since the *CFTR* gene was identified a large number of laboratories across the world have been characterizing the disease-associated mutations in the *CFTR* genes of their CF patient population and contributing their data to the Cystic Fibrosis Genetic Analysis Consortium. This data collection was originally established and coordinated by Dr Lap-Chee Tsui at the Hospital for Sick Children in Toronto. By 2007 more than 1500 mutations in the *CFTR* gene that are associated with CF disease had been identified.

What types of errors in the *CFTR* gene cause cystic fibrosis?

The errors in the *CFTR* gene that cause CF are called mutations. These can occur in a number of ways and these effects on CFTR protein function are summarized in Figure 13.4.

Deletions

The most common mutation in Britain, North America, and most of northern Europe is the deletion of one amino acid, phenylalanine, at position 508 of the protein (ΔF508). The effect of this mutation on the protein is to prevent the normal process of passage of the protein to the membrane of the cell (see Figure 13.4). CFTR protein builds up within the cell instead, where it cannot perform its usual functions. There are now many examples of other deletion mutations in the *CFTR* gene, which have a variety of effects depending on their size and location within the gene. Some remove large chunks of the gene so preventing the synthesis of any CFTR protein, others only remove a small amount of DNA but they too can have a dramatic effect on CFTR protein. The net result of a deletion mutation is usually a non-functional, truncated, or non-existent CFTR protein.

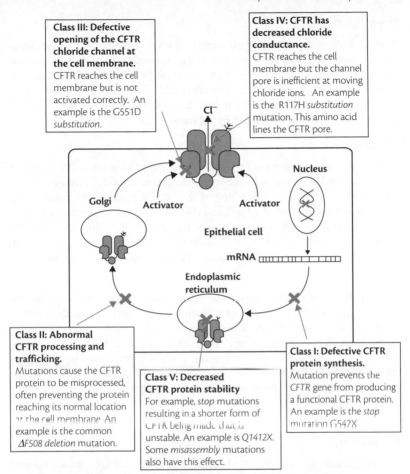

Class III: Defective opening of the CFTR chloride channel at the cell membrane. CFTR reaches the cell membrane but is not activated correctly. An example is the G551D *substitution*.

Class IV: CFTR has decreased chloride conductance. CFTR reaches the cell membrane but the channel pore is inefficient at moving chloride ions. An example is the R117H *substitution* mutation. This amino acid lines the CFTR pore.

Class II: Abnormal CFTR processing and trafficking. Mutations cause the CFTR protein to be misprocessed, often preventing the protein reaching its normal location at the cell membrane. An example is the common *ΔF508 deletion* mutation.

Class V: Decreased CFTR protein stability For example, *stop* mutations resulting in a shorter form of CFTR being made that is unstable. An example is Q1412X. Some *misassembly* mutations also have this effect.

Class I: Defective CFTR protein synthesis. Mutation prevents the *CFTR* gene from producing a functional CFTR protein. An example is the *stop* mutation G542X.

Figure 13.4 Mutations in the *CFTR* gene and how they alter function of the CFTR chloride channel. Two copies of the *CFTR* gene exist in the nucleus of every cell in the body. In specialized epithelial cells it is active and makes a message (shown as mRNA) that is translated into the CFTR protein. This is processed (correctly folded into a functional CFTR channel) in the endoplasmic reticulum and Golgi sub-compartments within the cell and then inserted into the cell membrane (the envelope that surrounds the cell) where it pumps chloride ions. Mutations in the *CFTR* gene can affect any part of this complex process. Five classes of mutation are shown which differ in how they impair CFTR function. Modified from Welsh, M. J., and Smith, A. E. (1993). 'Molecular mechanisms of CFTR chloride channel dysfunction in cystic fibrosis', *Cell*, 73, 12514 with revisions from Welsh, M., Ramsey, B., Accurso, F., and Cutting, G. R. (2001), 'The Molecular and Metabolic Basis of Inherited Disease', in C. R. Scriver, A. R. Beaudot, W. S. Sly, and D. Valle, eds, (New York: McGraw-Hill), pp. 5121–5188.

Stops

Another type of mutation, which occurs relatively frequently in some populations, is the alteration of a single coding unit within the DNA so that the protein synthesis machinery receives a signal to 'stop' rather than to put the next amino acid into the protein. The effect of this is to make a truncated protein rather than full-length CFTR and these short, part-proteins are usually unstable and non-functional, if they are made at all.

Substitutions

A frequent type of mutation in CFTR is the substitution of a single coding unit in the DNA, resulting in the wrong amino acid being inserted into the CFTR protein at that point. Many of the CFTR proteins with one wrong amino acid have been studied within cells. They usually reach the cell membrane and are correctly inserted into it, but then do not function correctly. Different amino acids have a wide range of biochemical properties that can greatly influence the three-dimensional structure and the activity of the whole CFTR protein.

A particularly interesting group of substitution mutations is those that alter specific amino acids in the transmembrane portions of CFTR (see Figure 13.4) and that interfere slightly with the normal passage of chloride across the cell membrane. These mutations have been found in some CF patients with milder disease, including normal pancreatic function, even when the other CF gene is the 'severe' *delta F508*. (Remember that mutations in both one's CF genes must be present before disease will manifest itself – having only one CF mutation results in being a carrier for the disease.)

Misassembly

The mechanism whereby the 6200 coding units of the *CFTR* gene are extracted from 190 000 total units in the gene is complex. Essentially, 27 segments of various lengths of coding units that make up the 6200 are extracted from a RNA copy of the whole *CFTR* gene and joined to each other. There are very precise signals built into the DNA units of the gene at the beginning and end of each of these 27 segments that cause the segments to become correctly joined together. Mutations in these signal regions can result in one or more of the 27 segments being left out, so that the message produced for the protein-making machinery is shorter than 6200 coding units. This usually means that normal CFTR is not made.

CFTR regulation

At the moment we understand very little about what actually regulates the activity of the *CFTR* gene and protein within the cell. Nor do we know what 'switches on' the gene in the cells where the CFTR protein is found. However, it is likely that as our hunt for disease-causing mutations in the *CFTR* gene moves out of the 6200 unit coding region, we will start finding parts of the DNA that control the gene. By drawing parallels with other genetic diseases, we expect to discover that some mutations occurring in these control regions cause the CFTR protein not to be produced at all or to be greatly reduced in some CF patients. The lack of the important CFTR protein within the specialized cells that normally express it then causes disease.

In terms of CFTR protein function, scientists have made their own classification of *CFTR* mutations, based on the properties of the resultant CFTR protein: class I mutations have no CFTR protein; class II have protein that is improperly processed and ends up in the wrong place in the cell, such as *ΔF508*; class III mutations generate CFTR proteins that get to the right place in the cell (the cell membrane) but do not function properly once they get there as they are improperly regulated; class IV mutations result in proteins that are correctly inserted into the cell membrane but have the wrong amino acids in the pore through which chloride ions are meant to pass out of the cell, so impeding this process; class V mutations are associated with reduced synthesis of functional CFTR protein.

CF modifier genes

Since the isolation of the *CFTR* gene and the start of the hunt for mutations associated with CF it has become clear that there are other genetic and non-genetic factors that influence disease severity. For example there is a wide variety of severity found in individuals who have two copies of the same mutation, for example *ΔF508*. Some of this variation can be accounted for by environmental factors, for example the age of diagnosis of CF: the earlier the disease is detected and rigorous treatments started, the better the clinical outcome. However, other genes are involved in determining the course of the disease and the hunt is on for what these genes might be. To date, at least two genes have been implicated as modifiers of lung disease, both of them involved in lung defence/repair and/or inflammation. There are likely to be other genes that contribute to the severity of other aspects of CF disease and to lung function.

FAQ

Do different mutations affect the severity of CF disease?

The answer to this question is not clear-cut. Though some mutations are more likely to be associated with severe disease than others, there are always exceptions. Thus, although $\Delta F508$ is generally regarded as a mutation that causes severe disease there are still many individuals who have two copies of the $\Delta F508$ mutation and have much milder disease, or for example have mild lung disease but severe intestinal disease. It does, however, seem to be the case that CF patients who carry two $\Delta F508$ *CFTR* genes are more likely to be pancreatic insufficient (that is to require enzyme supplements to help them digest their food) than are patients with a variety of other CF-associated mutations. There are a very few alterations or mutations of the CF gene which do generally appear to cause milder, though still significant, disease. As mentioned above, the existence of additional genetic modifiers of the CF phenotype and non-genetic contributing factors makes it hard to predict the disease course in any individual with known mutations in CFTR.

Note: Occasionally, when giving information to a CF patient about the particular mutations that they carry, a genetic counsellor may use what appears to be a code (e.g. see Figure 13.4). This code is in fact quite simple and works as follows. Every amino acid in the CFTR protein has a number that denotes its position in the protein chain. In addition there is a single-letter code to denote the particular chemical structure of the amino acid. When an error in the gene causes the wrong amino acid to be inserted into the protein chain at that point, this is described by a letter–number–letter shorthand. For example, quite a common mutation in the *CFTR* gene is called *G551D*, which means simply that at position 551 in the protein chain the normal glycine (code G) amino acid has been replaced by an aspartic acid (code D) amino acid.

In the same code, the letter X is read as a 'stop' signal by the machinery that joins together the amino acids in the protein. The common mutation *G542X* means that at position 542 the normal glycine (code G) amino acid has been replaced by a signal to stop adding amino acids to the protein chain. The terms 'ins' and 'del' simply denote the insertion of extra unwanted coding units or the deletion of essential coding until in the

CFTR gene. So *ins1154TC* means the insertion of a T and a C unit after the normal base 1154 in the *CFTR* message.

Does the inheritance of different mutations from each of the parents affect severity?

There is no good evidence for the inheritance of different mutations from each parent having a direct effect on disease severity. It has been difficult to collect data on a sufficient number of individuals with the same combination of two rarer mutations to rule out the effects of natural variation between individuals that has got nothing to do with the particular mutation in the CF gene. However, it would be generally true to say that there is as yet no substantial evidence for different combinations of mutations affecting disease severity. However, certain mutations that have relatively little effect on the CFTR protein can partially compensate for a mutation having a profound effect on the protein in the other *CFTR* gene of a CF patient.

Do different mutations require different treatments?

The answer to this question is no – at least not yet – as the current therapies for CF are irrespective of the mechanism by which *CFTR* malfunctions. It is possible that this might change at some time in the future (see below). Clearly patients with sufficient pancreatic function not to require enzyme supplements are spared this part of treatment. However, such patients (usually not carrying the ΔF508 mutation in both their *CFTR* genes) are in a minority and often progress to being pancreatic insufficient and hence require enzyme supplements as the disease proceeds. All other aspects of the treatment for CF will rather be tailored to treat the current clinical problems of the disease in an individual regardless of the mutations that he or she carries.

Do different mutations affect the outlook for future treatments by drugs or gene therapy?

The answer to this question depends on the type of treatment envisaged. Most of the current approaches to developing new treatments for CF are largely aimed at 'bypassing' the defective CFTR protein rather than actually correcting the mutant protein itself (see Chapter 12). If these approaches prove successful then the precise genetic cause of the failure to produce functional CFTR will not matter. However, other potential new treatments are tailored to correct the function of a specific mutation in CFTR. The most intensively studied is the $\Delta F508$ mutation and the development of treatments that would help the $\Delta F508$ protein to be properly folded and reach the cell membrane. However, this therapy would only be effective for individuals with at least one copy of the $\Delta F508$ mutation. This would include the majority of CF patients due to the high prevalence of this mutation. Another therapeutic route that is being investigated is the use of drugs to suppress the 'stop' mutations that occur in some CFTR proteins. This would obviously only be applicable to individuals carrying these mutations.

14

Genetic counselling in cystic fibrosis

Julian Forton

> ### ⮕ Key points
>
> ◆ Parents who already have a child with CF have a 1 in 4 chance of another child with CF in each pregnancy
>
> ◆ Diagnostic tests for CF can be done early in pregnancy (10–13 weeks) by a technique called chorionic villus sampling
>
> ◆ 95 per cent of men with CF are infertile but techniques are available to permit them to become fathers
>
> ◆ Advice on genetic risks (genetic counselling) is available for people who have CF in the family

Genetic counselling aims to provide detailed information to individuals who have a risk of producing children with a genetic disease, so that they are fully informed about the consequences of that disorder, the likelihood of their offspring being affected and the family-planning options that are available to them.

Parents of children with CF used to be limited to refraining from having further children or accepting a 1 in 4 chance of having another child with CF. Historically families tended to avoid having further children for fear of having another affected child.

Genetic counselling together with pre-natal testing, pre-implantation genetic diagnosis, carrier detection tests, and developments in assisted fertility for both men and women now provide many options in family planning for patients and families affected by CF.

There are four potential situations where genetic counselling for cystic fibrosis will be important to individuals planning a family:

1. Couples who already have a child with CF.

2. Couples with a family history of CF.

3. Adults who have CF.

4. The general population where parent carrier screening programmes or pre-natal testing during pregnancy is available.

The methods for genetic testing are described below, followed by the details of counselling for each of these situations.

Genetic testing

Mutation analysis

As outlined in the chapter on CF genetics, many different mutations of the *CFTR* gene may cause CF.

CF is the most common potentially lethal autosomal recessive disease among Caucasians, with a carrier frequency around 1 in 25 individuals and a prevalence of CF disease of 1 in 2500. In Hispanic–American people the carrier frequency is 1 in 46, which corresponds to a CF prevalence of around 1 in 8500. In African–American people the carrier frequency is 1 in 62 and the prevalence of CF is around 1 in 15 000: 1 in 25 000 Asian–American people have CF. The condition is extremely rare in Chinese people.

The frequency of specific CF mutations varies tremendously between ethnic groups. In Caucasians the *ΔF508* mutation is present on 70 per cent of all CF chromosomes. Across Europe there is a gradient of distribution for *ΔF508* with a higher incidence in northern countries such as those in Scandinavia compared with south-eastern countries such as Italy and Turkey.

In the Ashkenazi Jewish population the *ΔF508* mutation accounts for only 30 per cent of CF chromosomes and the most common mutation is *W1282X*. In African–American people *ΔF508* accounts for 48 per cent of CF chromosomes and in some Indian populations may account for just 19 per cent of CF chromosomes although it is generally closer to 50 per cent.

As mutation analysis of the CF gene has progressed it has become clear that certain genetic populations have a high frequency of mutations that are much rarer in other populations. This is clearly of importance when devising CF screening strategies for different genetic groups.

More than 1500 CFTR mutations and 200 sequence variants have been identified. The vast majority of these mutations are very rare and may only occur in one or two families. Data from laboratories around the world have identified collections of the most important mutations to use in screening of their populations. In the UK, using just four mutations ($\Delta F508$, $G551D$, $G542X$ and $621+1G>T$) will identify more than 80 per cent of all CF mutations. Extending up to the commercially available panel of 31 mutations will detect around 96 per cent of CF mutations. Even with extended panels, there will be occasions when mutations are not identified. However, in families with CF, genetic counselling can still be given even when the exact mutation cannot be identified. By using other markers on the chromosome which are reliably transmitted from parent to child, inheritance of CF chromosomes can be accurately followed from the affected relative down the family tree.

Methods of pre-natal diagnosis

Most methods of pre-natal diagnosis rely on obtaining some tissue from the baby which can then be tested for CF DNA mutations. Cells that originate from the baby can be obtained from the fluid in the womb surrounding the baby (the amniotic fluid), from the baby's blood as sampled from the umbilical cord, and from sampling the membranes surrounding the baby, known as the chorionic villi. All the procedures discussed have an acceptable low risk of interfering with the developing baby and have been used successfully in the pre-natal diagnosis of a variety of different genetic diseases.

Amniocentesis

This test is usually carried out between 16 and 18 weeks gestation and involves sampling the amniotic fluid. The procedure requires introduction of a thin needle into the mother's abdomen and into the fluid-filled amniotic sac that surrounds the baby. This is done with the guidance of ultrasound imaging. The procedure is performed under local anaesthetic and takes about half an hour. Amniocentesis has a small risk of miscarriage (1 per cent) and a small risk of premature birth (1 per cent).

The amniotic fluid that is obtained contains skin cells that the baby has shed and these can be harvested and grown (cultured) in the laboratory. When there are enough cells, DNA can be extracted and CF mutation analysis performed. Results from amniocentesis may take some days to return from the lab because of the need to culture the cells before doing the tests.

Fetal blood sampling

This is a newer technique and involves sampling blood from the baby. Blood is most easily drawn from the vessels in the umbilical cord, again by using a long thin needle and ultrasound guidance. This method is often used in the management of blood disorders such as thalassaemia or rhesus haemolytic disease where blood transfusions may also need to be given. It is a very complex procedure and requires a highly specialized team, and would generally only be used for genetic testing if other approaches are not possible or have not been successful. It can be used for rapid testing as sufficient cells for immediate DNA testing can be harvested. It carries a 1 per cent chance of miscarriage.

Chorionic villus sampling

Amniocentesis and fetal blood sampling are only useful at quite a late stage in pregnancy (16–18 weeks). At such a late stage, termination of the pregnancy is difficult both physically and psychologically for the mother. Chorionic villus sampling (CVS) can be performed from 10 weeks' gestation and the vast majority of pre-natal testing for CF is performed using this approach. The method involves removing a small piece of tissue from the membranes surrounding the baby. A thin, hollow tube is inserted into the womb through the birth canal and guided to the chorion using ultrasound imaging. A small piece of chorion about 2 mm wide is sucked into the tube and removed for testing. The same procedure may be performed through the wall of the abdomen, similar to amniocentesis.

Rapid results can be obtained from CVS without the need for cell culture – CVS therefore provides an early test with a rapid result. CVS carries a 1–2 per cent risk of miscarriage.

Ultrasound

Ultrasound is used to visualize the developing baby, placenta and structures of the womb during pregnancy. As well as being used for all the procedures outlined above, it is also routinely used in every pregnancy at between 20–22 weeks' gestation to screen for visible abnormalities in the developing baby. This is called the anomaly scan. Meconium ileus, the blockage of the bowel that occurs in some CF babies, may occasionally be detected on the anomaly scan, alerting the obstetrician to the possible diagnosis of CF. Its role in pre-natal testing for CF is limited but may support other tests suggesting the developing baby may have CF. It is non-invasive and carries no increased risk of miscarriage.

Pre-implantation genetic diagnosis for CF

Pre-implantation genetic diagnosis is an alternative to pre-natal diagnosis that enables diagnostic testing for a genetic disorder in an IVF (in vitro fertilization) embryo before it is implanted into the womb. The advantage of this approach is that parents with a high risk of a genetic disorder can have unaffected offspring without having to consider termination of pregnancy.

Embarking on this approach to achieving a healthy baby is a large commitment. First, both parents will need to be tested and counselled for their individual suitability. If accepted, the mother needs to take hormone treatment to ripen a number of eggs, have tests to assess when they are ripe and then under-go harvesting of the healthiest eggs by keyhole surgery. Five or six eggs are then fertilized in the laboratory with the partner's sperm. If the father has CF, the sperm will need to be harvested. Sperm may be retrieved by several methods. Epididymal sperm (see page 94) is usually collected either by micro-surgical epididymal sperm aspiration (MESA) under a general or local anaes-thetic or by percutaneous epididymal sperm aspiration (PESA) using a needle under local anaesthetic. PESA can be performed in the outpatient clinic but retrieves much smaller amounts of sperm and may need to be repeated during the course of a treatment. In cases where epididymal retrieval is unsuccessful, testicular excisional biopsy extraction (TESE) may be used where some tissue from the testis is removed and sperm harvested.

In the laboratory, a process called intracytoplasmic sperm injection (ICSI) is used where the sperm is actually injected into the egg. This gives better results than conventional in-vitro fertilization when using a small amount of sperm. After 48 hours the healthiest-looking embryos are selected and one or two cells are removed from each by micropipette. At this stage in the develop-ing embryo all the cells still have the individual capacity to grow into a fully formed baby. Removing two cells does not damage the embryo. DNA from these cells is used to test whether the embryo has CF. Embryos with no CF genes on screening are selected for implantation. The pregnancy rate per cycle is 20–25 per cent. The rate of misdiagnosis is between 1 and 5 per cent and so pre-natal testing by CVS after 10 weeks' gestation is advised.

Pre-implantation genetic diagnosis is not widely available and requires high-ly specialized expertise. Were it more freely available, there is no doubt that there are couples that would prefer this option to one of pre-natal testing in pregnancy with the option of termination. This group includes those couples who have had pre-natal diagnosis in the past, which may have resulted in a termination of an affected baby, and those who cannot accept termination of pregnancy either through religious or moral conviction.

Couples who already have a child with CF

The following facts would need to be communicated to a couple with a CF-affected child during a counselling session.

◆ The nature of CF, its morbidity, the prognosis and the burden for the child and family.

◆ The risk of having an affected child will be 1 in 4 for each pregnancy.

◆ The availability of accurate pre-natal diagnostic tests by chorionic villus sampling (CVS) at between 10 and 13 weeks' gestation, with results available within a few days. The risk of miscarriage from CVS is about 1 per cent above the pre-existing risk of any woman miscarrying after 10 weeks.

◆ Although not yet universally available, pre-implantation genetic diagnosis is an alternative to pre-natal testing, where couples are given the opportunity to have unaffected children without the need to consider termination. Couples undergo in vitro fertilization. Embryos generated in the test tube are genetically tested for CF mutations allowing implantation of an early CF-free embryo.

Attitudes towards having more children in families who already have a child with CF are changing, with up to 60 per cent of couples having subsequent offspring.

Acceptance of pre-natal testing and selective termination is a complex decision influenced by many factors. These include the severity of disease the couple have experienced with their first child, the perceived ability to cope with a second affected child, the influence and advice of the CF clinic team, religious convictions, the feeling that termination would send a negative message to their first child, and the timing of tests and whether the pregnancy can be kept private until results are clear.

The couple's experience of CF with their first child is likely to be one of the most important influences on decision-making. Parents of young children with CF will often have been given very encouraging advice about what the future holds in terms of prognosis and hopes of new treatments. Many children with CF identified through newborn screening will be asymptomatic during the time that their parents are considering having another child.

A nationally held register has shown that parents of young children with CF are less likely to have pre-natal tests and terminate a pregnancy compared with older parents with older children with CF, underlining the impression that perception of disease severity is likely to influence reproductive behaviour.

A couple's decision to pursue or terminate a pregnancy on the basis of pre-natal testing may well vary at different times in their lives. They may choose to terminate one pregnancy, then make the decision to continue with a second regardless of the outcome of pre-natal testing. Genetic counselling must therefore always be available.

Pre-natal screening is taken up by 70 per cent of couples, who either want to be prepared for another affected child or who intend to selectively terminate an affected pregnancy.

With the prognosis in CF difficult to forecast accurately, it is unsurprising that couples differ in their uptake of pre-natal diagnosis. Generally, attitudes towards pre-natal testing and selective termination of pregnancy are very positive in this group of parents, reinforcing the fact that many parents still perceive CF to be a severe disease.

Couples with a family history of CF

More and more relatives of people with CF have been seeking genetic counselling with their partners.

Table 14.1 overleaf summarizes the chance of being a CF carrier and the risk of having an affected child for different relatives in a family affected with CF, before any genetic testing.

For a couple who have family history of CF, both partners need to be assessed to see if they are CF carriers, before the chance of them having an affected child can be fully estimated.

The 'active cascade' screening programme implemented in the UK is a scheme where relatives of a person diagnosed with CF can be screened to see if they are carriers. The aim is to detect carrier couples where both partners are carriers, as these families have a 1 in 4 risk of having an affected child with their first pregnancy. Cascade screening should be highlighted to all parents with a new diagnosis of CF in the family. Families with an affected individual are generally very enthusiastic about contacting relatives to advise them of the availability of tests.

Table 14.1 The chance of being a CF carrier and the risk of having an affected child, for different relatives in a family affected with CF, *before* any genetic testing is performed (UK data)

Relationship to person with CF	Chance of being a carrier	Risk of having a child with CF with an *untested* partner
Parents	100%	1 in 4
Person with CF	100%	1 in 50
Parent remarries	100%	1 in 100
Child of women with CF	100%	1 in 100
Brother or sister	2 in 3	1 in 150
Aunt or uncle	1 in 2	1 in 200
Grandparent	1 in 2	1 in 200
First cousin	1 in 4	1 in 400
Second cousin	1 in 8	1 in 800

From the CF Trust factsheet on the family cascade screening programme for cystic fibrosis.

In cascade screening, DNA is obtained using a simple mouthwash test to collect cheek cells. No blood test is required. Both partners are tested for the common mutations accounting for approximately 90 per cent of CF mutations. In addition, the specific mutations carried by the affected relative should be tested for in the partner with the relative on their side of the family.

If the CF mutations in the relative are not known, or cannot be identified because they are very rare mutations, testing for carrier status may be more complicated but is still usually possible. This is achieved by identifying other genetic markers of the chromosome carrying the CF gene in the affected relative, and working through the family tree to see whether this chromosome has been passed on.

If both partners are positive for a CF mutation the risk of an affected child is 1 in 4 and genetic counselling should be offered, with reference to the availability of pre-natal diagnosis and pre-implantation genetic screening. If the partner with the affected relative is positive but their partner is negative, the risk of an affected child is in the region of 1 in 1000, and reassurance of low risk can be given. If the partner with the affected relative is negative but their partner is positive, the risk is lower at around 1 in 2000, and if both partners are negative, the risk is in the region of 1 in 250 000. These statistics are summarized in Table 14.2.

For a CF carrier with an untested partner the risk of having an affected child is 1 in 100.

Table 14.2 The chance of having a child with CF for a couple after testing

Results	Risk of having a child with CF	Action
Both partners are carriers	1 in 4	Genetic counselling. Options are discussed including tests and support available in current and future pregnancies.
Relative carrier/partner negative	1 in 1000	Low risk. Reassurance given. Tests not routinely offered in pregnancy. Check offspring if sickly.
Relative negative/partner positive	1 in 2000	Low risk. Reassurance given. Tests not routinely offered in pregnancy. Check offspring if sickly.
Both partners negative	Less than 1 in 250 000	Strong reassurance

From the CF Trust factsheet on the family cascade screening programme for cystic fibrosis.

Adults who have CF

With increasing survival, almost 50 per cent of patients with CF are now in the adult population and are keen to have children. One study showed that 78 per cent of men with CF wanted to have children irrespective of disease severity.

Men with CF

In counselling men with CF regarding assisted fertility the following points need to be clarified:

- 95 per cent of men with CF are infertile.

- Sperm production in the testes is likely to be normal but ejaculate will not contain sperm because of the absence of the vas deferens.

- Sperm aspiration coupled with IVF techniques can result in successful pregnancy.

- The child will definitely be a CF carrier.

- The partner must be tested for CF mutations. If common mutations are excluded, there is still a risk of around 1 in 500 that the child will be affected by CF. Pre-implantation genetic diagnosis and pre-natal testing with potential for selective termination should therefore be considered.

- Reduced life expectancy for the father should be discussed frankly and honestly with both partners. The likelihood of the mother having to care for both her partner and her child later in life must be considered in the decision-making process.

Ninety-five per cent of men with CF are infertile because the male genital ducts are blocked or absent. This is called congenital bilateral absence of the vas deferens (CBAVD). The testes continue to function and produce sperm, but they are trapped and are not present in ejaculate.

Some men have isolated CBAVD without clinical symptoms of CF. With advances in the genetic understanding of CF it has become clear that there is genetic overlap between these two conditions. In one study 60 per cent of men with CBAVD carried one CF mutation, 20 per cent carried two mutations and 20 per cent carried no detectable mutations. Isolated CBAVD may be associated with lower expression levels of normal CFTR which are still sufficient to prevent the classic manifestations of CF.

Men with CF have the potential to be genetic fathers through the use of techniques for sperm retrieval from the epididymis or testis itself (see above). In men with isolated CBAVD, sperm are normal and retrieval methods have been largely successful. Less evidence is available for men with CF whose sperm may not always be normal. A small study from the USA reported a 60 per cent success in retrieval and fertilization of the egg using ICSI, with a 50 per cent success in achieving a live birth. Success may be particularly difficult with more severe CF mutations including the common $\Delta F508$ mutation.

Fertility treatment for men with CF in the UK amounts to a handful in each centre but is likely to increase with improvements in technology and an increase in referrals.

Pregnancy in women with CF

Two thirds of women with cystic fibrosis are able to become pregnant spontaneously and therefore, unlike men with CF, do not always require the input of reproductive specialists.

This means that counselling women with CF regarding both contraception and the possibility of having a child should be proactive and take place in good time, so that the mother-to-be is fully informed of the consequences of CF in pregnancy, the impact it may have on her health and the health of her child, and the tests that can be done to minimize the risk of the couple's child being affected by CF.

In counselling women with CF regarding pregnancy the following points need to be clarified:

◆ Two-thirds of women with CF are able to become pregnant spontaneously.

◆ Becoming pregnant does increase illness.

◆ Having a baby does not impact on the mother's long-term survival.

◆ Children of mothers with CF are more often premature and of low birth-weight, particularly if the mother has poor lung function.

◆ All children will be CF carriers. It is therefore imperative that the father is tested to see if he is a carrier. If common mutations are excluded in the father, there is still a risk of around 1 in 500 that the child will be affected by CF. Pre-implantation genetic diagnosis and pre-natal testing with potential for selective termination should therefore be considered.

◆ The severity of the woman's CF and her ability to cope with a baby would dominate decisions on the wisdom of undertaking a pregnancy.

◆ Reduced life expectancy for the mother should be discussed frankly and honestly with both partners. This means the partner will eventually have sole responsibility for the child. The loss of a mother may have significant psychological and behavioural consequences for the child.

Many of the physiological effects of pregnancy may theoretically impact negatively on maternal health, including pressure on the lungs from the enlarging uterus, difficulty doing normal physiotherapy, an increase in gastric reflux and relative immunosuppression with more chest infections.

Becoming pregnant with CF does appear to increase illness. Patients have an increased requirement for intravenous and nebulized antibiotics, spend more days in hospital, are more likely to develop CF-related diabetes and often need a more aggressive approach to nutrition with some periods of intravenous feeding.

The possibility that a woman with CF may become very unwell or even die in pregnancy is still a reality, and those with severe or unstable disease should be counselled carefully regarding the wisdom of such an undertaking. Nevertheless, studies have shown that women with CF can often safely become pregnant and deliver healthy children. Becoming pregnant does not appear to affect long-term survival in women with CF, even for women with severe lung function impairment (forced expiratory volume (FEV) in one second of less than 40 per cent). It is not possible to predict which women with CF will tolerate pregnancy well and all pregnancies should therefore be followed closely at a specialist centre.

Community-wide CF carrier screening

Most children born with cystic fibrosis are born to parents with no family history of CF.

These families will therefore not be detected by cascade screening as outlined above and the choices available through genetic counselling can not be provided for their first affected child with CF.

Possible approaches to detecting these carrier couples include pre-conception screening in primary care or pre-natal carrier testing in early pregnancy. A programme of couple testing offered in the early pre-natal period implemented in Edinburgh has resulted in a halving of the incidence of CF in this region. Uptake of pre-natal CF carrier screening was around 80 per cent. Interestingly a couple's reproductive plans are not always altered on the basis of test results.

15

Survival

Cystic fibrosis is a life-shortening disease. It is not possible to give an estimate of how long babies with CF born today will live but it is not unreasonable to expect them to live into their 40s or 50s. Life for a baby born today is very different from 30 years ago in all sorts of ways including treatment for cystic fibrosis. Specialist cystic fibrosis centres were few and far between then; there was no surveillance with regular cough swabs, and antibiotics were less sophisticated. The importance of good nutrition was not understood and individuals were still on low-fat rather than high-fat diets. Pancreatic enzymes were not coated to protect them from stomach acid, and other drugs such as nebulized antibiotics and DNase were not available.

It is not surprising that the expectation is that today's children will do very much better than their predecessors, even without the new therapies which are likely to become available during their lifetime. The goal is to keep them as well as possible for as long as possible so that they are in the best condition to benefit from the new treatments as they come along.

Appendix 1

Further reading

Comeau AM, Accurso FJ, White TB, Campbell PW 3rd, Hoffman G, Parad RB, Wilfond BS, Rosenfeld M, Sontag MK, Massie J, Farrell PM, O'Sullivan BP. Guidelines for implementation of cystic fibrosis newborn screening programs: Cystic Fibrosis Foundation workshop report. *Pediatrics* 2007; 119(2):e495–518.

Davies JC, Alton EW. Airway gene therapy. *Advances in Genetics* 2005; 54: 291–314.

Davies JC, Alton EW, Bush A. Cystic fibrosis. *British Medical Journal* 2007; 5; 335(7632): 1255–1259 (Subject review).

Dodge JA, Lewis PA, Stanton M, Wilsher J. Cystic fibrosis mortality and survival in the UK: 1947–2003. *European Respiratory Journal* 2007; 29:522–526.

Dodge JA, Turck D. Cystic fibrosis: nutritional consequences and management. *Best Practice and Research in Clinical Gastroenterology* 2006; 20(3):531 516.

Elborn S. How can we prevent multisystem complications of cystic fibrosis? *Seminars in Respiratory Critical Care Medicine* 2007; 28(3):303–311 (Subject review).

Elston C, Geddes D. Inflammation in cystic fibrosis – when and why? Friend or foe? *Seminars in Respiratory Critical Care Medicine* 2007; 28(3):286–294 (Subject review).

Gibson RL, Burns JL, Ramsey BW. Pathophysiology and management of pulmonary infections in cystic fibrosis. *American Journal of Respiratory Critical Care Medicine* 2003; 168:918–915.

Glasscoe CA, Quittner AL. Psychological interventions for cystic fibrosis. *Cochrane Database System Review* 2003; 3:CD003148.

Hink H, Schellhase D.Transitioning families to adult cystic fibrosis care. *Journal for Specialists in Pediatric Nursing* 2006; 11(4):260–263 (Subject review).

Kerem E, Conway S, Elborn S, Heijerman H; Consensus Committee. Standards of care for patients with cystic fibrosis: a European consensus. *Journal of Cystic Fibrosis* 2005; 4:7–26.

Madge S.Growing up and growing older with cystic fibrosis. *Journal of the Royal Society of Medicine* 2006; 99(Suppl. 46):23–26 (Subject review).

Main E, Prasad A, Schans C. Conventional chest physiotherapy compared to other airway clearance techniques for cystic fibrosis. *Cochrane Database System Review* 2005; 25(1):CD002011 (Subject review).

Marks JH. Airway clearance devices in cystic fibrosis. *Paediatric Respiratory Reviews* 2007; 8(1):17–23 (Subject review).

Milla CE. Nutrition and lung disease in cystic fibrosis. *Clinics in Chest Medicdine* 2007; 28(2):319–330 (Subject review).

Minasian C, McCullagh A, Bush A. Cystic fibrosis in neonates and infants. *Early Human Develpoment* 2005; 81(12):997–1004 (Subject review).

Saeed Z, Wojewodka G, Marion D, Guilbault C, Radzioch D. Novel pharmaceutical approaches for treating patients with cystic fibrosis. *Current Pharmaceutical Design* 2007; 13(31):3252–3263 (Subject review).

Scriver CR, Beaudot AR, Sly WS, Valle D (eds). *The Molecular Basis of Inherited Disease.* New York: McGraw Hill, 2001, pp. 5121–5158.

Strachan T, Read AP. *Human Molecular Genetics,* 3rd edn. London, New York: Garland Science, 2003.

Sueblinvong V, Whittaker LA. Fertility and pregnancy: common concerns of the aging cystic fibrosis population. *Clinics in Chest Medicine* 2007; 28(2):433–443 (Subject review).

Webb AK, Jones AW, Dodd ME. Transition from paediatric to adult care: problems that arise in the adult cystic fibrosis clinic. *Journal of the Royal Society of Medicine* 2001; 94(Suppl. 40):8–11 (Subject review).

Wicks E. Cystic fibrosis. *British Medical Journal* 2007; 334:1270–1271.

Williams, PD. The well sibling's perspective. In: Blubond-Cangner M, Lask B, Angst DB, *Psychosocial Aspects of Cystic Fibrosis* (2001). New York: Arnold Publishers.

Appendix 2

Cystic fibrosis associations

Argentina

Associación Argentina de Lucha
contra la Enfermedad Fibroquisitica
del Pancreas
Pueyrredon
1895 – 1'B 1119
Buenos Aires
Website: www.fipan.org.ar

Australia

Cystic Fibrosis Australia (CFA)
PO Box 254
North Ryde NSW 1670
Australia
Email.
general@cysticfibrosisaus tralia.org.au
Website: www.cysticfibrosis.org.au

Austria

Cystische Fibrose Hilfe
Österreich
Hanuschgasse 1
2540 Bad Vöslau
Austria
Email: office@cf-austria.at
Website: www.cf-austria.at

Belgium

Association Belge de Lutte
Contre La Mucoviscidose (ABLM)
Ave Joseph Borlé 12
1160 Brussels
Belgium
Email: info@muco.be
Website: www.muco.be

Brazil

Associação Brasileira de Assistência
à Mucoviscidose
R. João Negrão, 539 – Conj. 03
Curitiba/PR
Cx. Postal 19342
CEP 80251–970
Brazil
Website: www.abram.org.br

Bulgaria

State University Hospital
Alexandrovska Pediatric Clinic
Georgi Soffiisky str.
1431 Sofia
Bulgaria

Canada

Cystic Fibrosis Foundation
Suite 601
2221 Yonge Street
Toronto, Ont.
Canada M4S 2B4
Email: info@cysticfibrosis.ca
Website: www.cysticfibrosis.ca

Chile

Corp. Para la Fibrosis Quistica del
Pancreas
La Canada 6505 (i)
La Reina Santiago
Chile

Columbia

Fundacion Colombiana de Fibrosis
Quistica
D. Vladimiro Camacho
Apartado Aereo 2889
Santafe de Bogota
Colombia

Costa Rica

Asociación Costarricense de FQ
Hospital Nacional de Niños
PO 357–1002
Paseo de los Estudiantes
San José
Costa Rica

Cuba

Comision Cubana de
Fibrosis Quistica
Hospital Pediatrico JM Marquez
Ave. 31 esq.a 76, CP 11400
Municipio Marianao

Ciudad Habana
Cuba
Email: rojo@informed.sld.cu

Czech Republic

Klub Nemocných Cystickou
Fibrózou, o.s.
Kudrnova 22/95
150 18 Praha 5
Czech Republic
Email: info@cfklub.cz
Website: www.cfklub.cz

Denmark

Danish Cystic Fibrosis Association
Hyrdebakken 246
DK-8800 Viborg
Denmark
Email: hwt@cff.dk
Website: www.cystikfibrose.dk

Ecuador

Fundacion Ecuatoriana de Fibrosis
Quistica
Ciudadela Alborada Decima Etapa
Manzana 304 Villa Diez
Guayaquil
Ecuador
Email: jbernous@teleconet.net

El Salvador

Fundación Contra la Fibrosis Quística
Hospital Nacional de Niños
Benjamín Bloom
Boulevard Los Héroes
San Salvador
El Salvador
Website:
www.fundacionfibrosisquistica.org

France

Association Française de Lutte
contre la Mucoviscidose
181 Rue de Tolbiac
75013 Paris
France
Email: info@vaincrelamuco.org
www.vaincrelamuco.org

Germany

Mukoviszidose e.V.
In den Dauen 6
53117 Bonn
Germany
Email: info@mukoviszidose-ev.de
www.mukoviszidose-ev.de

Greece

Hellenic Cystic Fibrosis Association
Parashou & Papathymiou Str. 6
Athens 11475
Greece
Email: webmaster@hcfa.gr
Website: www.hcfa.gr

Hungary

Cystic Fibrosis Foundation
H 1124 Burok-u 15
Budapest
Hungary
Email: holicscf@matavnet.hu

Iceland

Cystic Fibrosis Association of Iceland
Newborn Intensive Care University
Barnaspitali Hringsins
Landspitalinn v/Baronsstig
101 Reykjavik
Iceland
Email: hordurb@landspitali.is

Ireland

Cystic Fibrosis Association of Ireland
Cystic Fibrosis House
24 Lower Rathmines Road
Dublin 6
Ireland
Website: www.cfireland.ie

Israel

Israel Cystic Fibrosis Association
79 Krinitzy st.
Ramat Gan
Israel 52423
Email: C.F.@classnet.co.il
Website: www.cf.org.il

Italy

Lega Italiana Fibrosi Cistica (LIFC)
Via San Vittore 39
20123 Milano
Italy
Website: www.fibrosicistica.it

Netherlands

Dutch Cystic Fibrosis Foundation
Dr A. Schweitzerweg 3
3744 MG Baarn
Netherlands
Email: info@ncfs.nl
Website: www.ncfs.nl

New Zealand

Cystic Fibrosis Association of
New Zealand
62 Riccarton Rd
PO Box 8241
Christchurch
New Zealand
Website: www.cfnz.org.nz

Norway

Norwegian Cystic Fibrosis
Association
Postboks 4568, Nydalen
0404 Oslo
Norway
Website: www.cfnorge.no

Poland

Polish Society Against Cystic
Fibrosis
ul. M.C. Sklodowskiej 2
34–700 Rabka Zdroj
Poland
Website: www.ptwm.org.pl

Portugal

Associacao Portuguesa de Fibrose
Quistica
Rua Mouzinho de Albuquerque 45
4400–231 Vila Nova Gaia
Portugal
Website: www.apfq.pt

Romania

Romanian CF Association
Str. Gh. Doja nr. 14
1900 Timisoara
Romania
Email: cp-bega@mailsoros.tm.ro

Slovak Republic

Klub Cystickej Fibrózy
Lofflerova 2
040 01 Kosice
Slovak Republic
Website: www.klubcf.sk

South Africa

National Cystic Fibrosis Association
PO Box 145691
Bracken Gardens 1452
Alberton
South Africa
Email: cfa@iafrica.com
Website: www.isisa.co.za/isisa/cystic

Spain

Federación Española de FQ
C/Duque de Gaeta 56 – pta. 14
46022 Valencia
Spain
Website: fqfederacion@fibrosis.org

Sweden

Swedish Cystic Fibrosis Association
Kålsängsgränd 10 D
SE-753 19 Uppsala
Sweden
Website: www.rfcf.se

Switzerland

Schweizerische Gesellschaft für
Cystische Fibrose (CFCH)
Postgasse 17, Postfach 686
CH-3000 Bern 8
Switzerland
Website: www.cfch.ch

Turkey

Pediatric Respiratory Disease
Association
Hacettepe University
Ankara 06100
Turkey
Website: www.pediatri.hacettepe.
edu.tr

United Kingdom

Cystic Fibrosis Research Trust
11 London Road
Bromley
Kent BR1 1BY
United Kingdom
Email: enquiries@cftrust.org.uk
Website: www.cftrust.org.uk

United States

Cystic Fibrosis Foundation
CFF 6931 Arlington Road
Bethesda, MD 20814
United States
Email: info@cff.org
Website: www.cff.org

Appendix 3

Glossary

acidosis — condition resulting from accumulation of acid or depletion of the alkaline (bicarbonate) reserves in the blood or body tissues.

aerosols — medications given by inhalation. In CF antibiotics, bronchodilators, saline, and Dornase alpha (DNase) are given this way.

alleles — the two forms of the same gene coexisting in the same cell, one being inherited from each of the parents.

alveoli — tiny, air-filled sacs in the lung tissue.

aspergillosis — inflammatory reaction to infection by the fungus *Aspergillus fumigatus*.

autosome — all chromosomes other than the sex chromosomes.

bacteria — micro-organisms (e.g. *Staphylococcus*, *Pseudomonas*), some of which may invade healthy tissues, others only damaged tissue, to cause infections. Some bacteria, e.g. the *Bacillus coli* of the large bowel, cause no infection and are in fact necessary for health.

bronchiectasis — a state of permanent abnormal widening of the bronchial walls, often because of infections and ball–valve phenomena which result in poor drainage of infected mucus.

bronchioles — small bronchi.

bronchoalveolar lavage — a technique where during a bronchoscopy fluid is passed down into the small airways and airspaces and then sucked up again through the bronchoscope. Used to identify infection in areas of the lung.

bronchodilator — a substance capable of relieving bronchospasm.

bronchoscopy — an investigation where a small camera is passed down the airways to examine them and to collect airway secretions.

bronchospasm — a reversible muscular contraction of the bronchi.

bronchus (plural bronchi) — a major branch of the airways.

carrier — an individual who has inherited a particular defective form of a recessive gene from one of his parents, but a normal form from the other. He thus 'carries' the defective gene, but suffers no ill effects from it.

centile chart — a chart which divides height or weight at any age into hundredths (percentiles) so, for example, 50 normal children in every 100 are above the 50th centile and 50 children are below; 97 children are above the 3rd centile and only 3 below.

cholecystitis — inflammation of the gallbladder, often associated with gallstones.

chromosomes — the structures within each cell that contain the genetic material.

cilia — minute mobile, hair-like processes projecting from the outer surface of a cell. The airways are lined with ciliated cells.

cirrhosis — fibrosis of the liver, interfering with the passage of blood from the intestine through liver cells.

coeliac disease — an inability to digest wheat proteins.

consanguinity — inbreeding between genetically related members of the same family.

cystic fibrosis transmembrane conductance regulator (CFTR) — the protein made by the CF gene. It is thought to regulate movements of charged salt molecules across cell membranes.

ΔF508 — the common mutation found in 70 per cent of CF genes in northern Europe and North America. It is caused by the loss of three bases in the DNA resulting in the absence of the amino acid phenylalanine at position 508 in the protein.

diploid — cells carrying two sets of genetic information.

DNA (deoxyribonucleic acid) — the major component of the genetic material. The biological molecule that codes for all the information needed to construct a human being from a single fertilized egg.

dominant — a gene, the effects of which are not masked by the presence of its normal counterpart in the same cell.

electrolytes — the different ions in fluid, e.g. sodium, potassium.

emphysema — permanent overdistension of the alveoli in the lung.

endocrine glands — a gland which discharges secretions directly into the bloodstream, e.g. insulin and glucagon from the pancreas.

enema — injection of liquid into the rectum.

enzyme — a protein which acts as a catalyst in a reaction, e.g. to break down a complex molecule.

epididymus — the first, coiled part of the duct system that takes sperm from the testis to the penis. The more distal duct is called the vas deferens.

exocrine gland — a gland that passes its secretions through ducts, e.g. trypsin and lipase from the pancreas. (The pancreas is both an exocrine and an endocrine gland.)

fibrosis — the replacement of normal tissue with scar tissue, e.g. in the pancreas.

genes — coding regions of DNA.

genome — all the genetic information of an individual.

haemoptysis — the coughing of blood.

haploid — cells carrying one set of genetic information (i.e. eggs and sperm).

heart–lung transplants — replacement of heart and lungs of a CF patient with those of an organ donor.

heterozygote — an individual who has inherited different forms of a particular gene from both parents.

homozygote — an individual who has inherited identical forms of a particular gene from both parents.

hormones — specific substances produced in endocrine glands (see above) that are secreted into the blood and are carried to all parts of the body. Hormones are quick-acting, required in very small amounts, and have a wide range of effects on body biochemistry.

ileostomy — the bringing of a loop of ileum to open on to the anterior abdominal wall to allow bowel contents to be passed.

ileus — literally, a disorder of motility of the ileum, resulting in the contents not being propelled towards the colon. In meconium ileus, contents are not propelled because of the tenacious meconium.

immunosuppressant (anti-rejection) drugs — drugs that suppress the natural immunological response of the body to reject foreign tissues and proteins.

intravenous — given directly into a vein.

intussusception — a pathological process in which a section of the small intestine folds into the adjoining region of downstream bowel, endangering its blood supply.

in vitro fertilization — fertilization of an egg by a sperm in a test tube in the laboratory.

ion — an electrically charged atom or molecule.

malabsorption — inability to absorb food normally in intestines due to poor digestion.

MCT oil — oil containing medium-chain triglycerides. These can be absorbed directly into the bloodstream from the intestine.

meconium — the first dark-green stools of the newborn.

meconium ileus — an obstruction of the small intestine at birth.

meiosis — the cell division process by which haploid cells are made from diploid ones.

messenger RNA — copied from DNA by transcription, this molecule is the blueprint for translation of the genetic information into biologically useful molecules, proteins.

metabolism — the set of chemical reactions that convert food to energy to maintain life.

mucolytic — a substance capable of thinning mucus. It may do this by increasing the water content of the mucus or by breaking chemical bonds between sulphur and hydrogen.

mutation — the occurrence of a spontaneous abnormality in a gene that is not found in the genes of the parent's cells.

nasal polyp — a growth resulting from the heaping up of mucous membrane in the nasal passages. Common in older children with CF.

nebulizer — a machine which converts a liquid to a fine spray (aerosol) which can be inhaled.

organ rejection — loss of function of donor organs due to the new host's immunological response to them.

pathogenesis — the evolution of the abnormal (pathological) changes of a disease process.

peritonitis — an acute inflammation of the peritoneum.

pneumothorax — air trapped between the outside (pleural) surface of the lung and the chest wall. This splints the lung and prevents its normal movement during breathing. In CF it would occur with the rupture of over-distended (emphysematous) alveoli. Removal of the air by a needle attached to an under-water drain may be necessary.

proximal bowel — the section of bowel closer to the mouth (**distal bowel** is the bowel section further from the mouth, i.e. closer to the anus).

recessive — a gene, the effects of which are masked by the present of its normal counterpart in the same cell.

recombination — the physical process by which new combinations of genes are made by shuffling of the genetic information prior to cell division.

spirometer — an instrument for measuring the air breathed into and out of the lungs.

sputum — phlegm coughed up from the airway passages.

steatorrhoea — literally, fatty diarrhoea. Recognized by pale, bulky, foul-smelling stools.

steroids — a group of substances that can be natural or artificial and which have a wide range of effects when given as medicines, including suppression of immunological responses.

varices — dilated veins.

vas deferens — the terminal part of the duct system that carries sperm from the testis to the penis.

X-linked — a gene on the X chromosome.

Index